How to get your back pain....

..*so it stays away*

ISBN: 0-646-37645-4
Author and publisher: Dr Graeme Blennerhassett
Cover design: Dr Graeme Blennerhassett and Nina Sanadze
Printed by: Australian Print Group, Maryborough, Australia
For distributors: **www.blcc.com.au**
To contact author/publisher: **www.blcc.com.au**
Bulk book orders: **www.blcc.com.au**

Some images used herein were obtained from MSI's Masterclips™ and Masterphotos™ Premium Image Collection, 1895 San Francisco Blvd. East, San Rafael, CA 94901-5506, USA

Disclaimer

1.   This book aims to give an overview for lay-people. As such, simplifications and generalisations are sometimes made.

2.   The book is for information purposes only. All spinal problems require professional diagnoses and management, not self diagnoses and management after reading a book. People with spinal problems should seek specific advice from a qualified health care provider. No responsibility is taken for anyone ignoring this advice.

3.   The advice given in this book will not work for everyone. Some back pain cannot be relieved. No results are guaranteed

Contents

DEDICATIONS

Extreme thanks is given to the following people who have helped develop this book and the ideas that it contains.

Dr. Dean Lines, who taught me the value of accurate testing of muscle function.

Dr. A.L. (Roy) Logan (dec.), who introduced a whole new common sense, biomechanically sound method of practice.

Dr. Gary Vagg, my valued friend who taught me many important aspects of practice, and was the first person to take care of my own spine really well.

Dr. Ray Broome, who gave me my first full appreciation of the principles of adjusting.

Dr. Sergio Carlie, owner of Quantum Workhealth, through which I learned much about communication and injury prevention.

Dr. Damian Darby, a very skilful chiropractor who takes wonderful care of my own spine.

Dr. Chris Barham, who opened my mind a bit more allowing me to give this book a heart and soul.

Dr. Daryl Ansell for his excellent feedback and support

My reviewers: Mandy Allen, Raan Carley, Don Petersen, Dr. Brian Kelly, Brian Clark, Dr. Daryl Smith

Joanne Eastman for some important suggestions.

Introduction

Who should read this book?

This book will provide answers and solutions for both those who have a back problem, those who want to avoid back problems, and those who want to be healthier.

Why read this book?

Patients face a real minefield when they seek care. They have little way of knowing whether the care they receive is sensible, or merely painting over rust dooming them to further problems years ahead.

Lets look at what happens

Take your sore back to ten different "experts" and you will likely get ten different diagnoses. Each will treat you a bit differently. Some will make it feel better, some seem to fix the problem, but the pain always seems to come back.

Why does this happen?

Firstly, spinal problems are usually a lot more complicated than simplistic explanations like "a bone out" or "a muscular problem" suggest.

Secondly, each profession tends to focus on their own area of expertise. Some practitioners, figuratively speaking, do not see the forest for the trees.

Finally, common sense and logic often get pushed aside in favor of sacred cows, vested interests and professional arrogance.

Where does this put the patients?

Unfortunately, not in a very good position. This author so frequently hears and sees "horror stories": patients getting inappropriate care and being brainwashed with misinformation.

What can a patient do?

Without knowledge, patients are at the mercy of any practitioner that appears credible or has a convincing story. All they can really go by is what makes them feel good. This can be very miss-leading.

With knowledge a patient is in a far better position to ask the right questions and get the right care.

The author presents some guidelines on how a spine should be cared for. While not perfect (they are undergoing continuing evolution) they do seem to be consistent with known facts and logic, and at least provide some guidelines that can be used for comparison.

Because all problems with a spine are different, and there is always the potential for something nasty to be present, readers with a spinal problem should always seek the help of a competent professional. No responsibility is taken for anyone ignoring this advice.

Chapter One

The parts and workings of a spine

Spine from the side

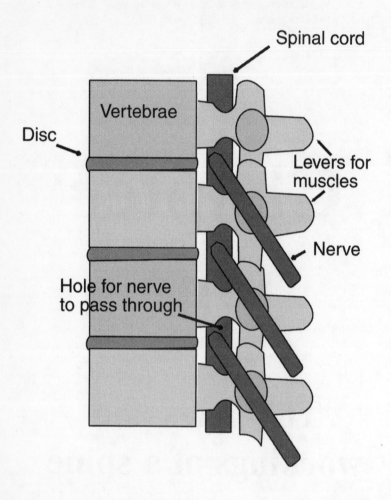

Spinal cord

Vertebrae

Disc

Levers for muscles

Nerve

Hole for nerve to pass through

Vertebrae

The spine has a column of bones called vertebrae.

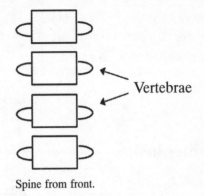

Vertebrae

Spine from front.

Discs

Most vertebrae are separated by pads called discs. The discs have an outside casing like a car tyre, and are filled with jelly (the jelly becomes solid as one gets older). The discs act as shock absorbers and allow movement.

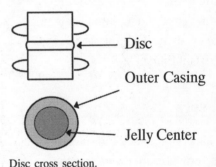

Disc

Outer Casing

Jelly Center

Disc cross section.

The Arch

At the rear of the vertebrae are bony arches. With the vertebrae as a column, the arches form a tube which houses and protects the spinal cord.

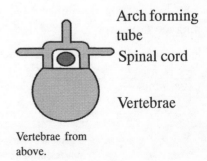

Arch forming tube

Spinal cord

Vertebrae

Vertebrae from above.

Holes for Nerves

There are grooves in the arches that form tunnels for the individual nerves to come out.

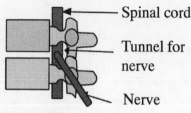

Spinal cord

Tunnel for nerve

Nerve

Spine from side.

Sliding Joints

At the rear of the vertebrae are the small sliding joints that help guide the movement of the spine. Their sliding surfaces are covered by a slippery wear resistant lining.

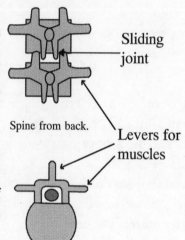

Sliding joint

Spine from back.

Levers for muscles

Levers

Poking out the back and sides of the vertebrae are levers that the muscles attach to.

Part of spine from above.

Ligaments

Between the vertebrae are bands of tough fibre called ligaments. They are loose enough to allow normal movement, but stop the spine bending too far.

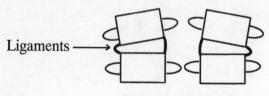

Ligaments ⟶

Ligaments restricting the movement of vertebrae.

Muscles

Muscles move bones by pulling on them. Attached to the spine are long muscles that support the spine and help make movements such as bending and twisting. Between close vertebrae there are short muscles. Although they help produce overall movement such as bending, they are more important as stabilisers for individual joints and to ensure that each joint moves evenly.

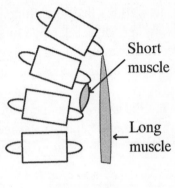

Short muscle

Long muscle

Short and long muscles.

Normal Movement

Movement should be smooth and even. For a spine to bend, each individual joint should move a little bit and share the work.

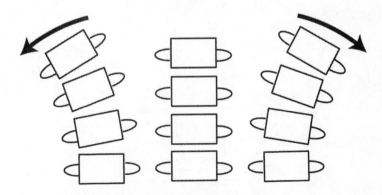

Normal smooth even movement.

Pain

Pain is a warning that something is wrong. Sensors throughout the body may detect damage or some abnormality, then send an electrical message along a nerve to the brain. The brain should receive the message and do something to correct the problem.

It is a bit like having a temperature sensor in a car engine detect over-heating and send a message to the dash board warning light. The driver would stop the car and have the problem fixed.

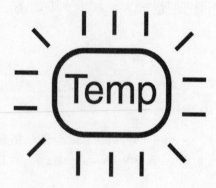

Pain is natures warning system.

Chapter Two

What happens to the spine to make it deteriorate and become sore

What happens to the spine to make it deteriorate and become sore

The basic process

Most problems with a spine follow basically the same pattern. An initial injury* upsets the balance and movement of the spine. This places abnormal stress and load on most, if not all, the parts. Parts affected include the muscles, bones, ligaments and nervous system. Because of the abnormal stress and load the parts deteriorate and may eventually 'give out'. Here are the details of what happens.

Initial injury

The joints of a spine should be balanced and move freely. If a spinal joint is injured the surrounding small muscles will pull tight to form a natural immobilising splint while the damage heals. Other joints close to the injured joint may help by doing a little bit extra work.

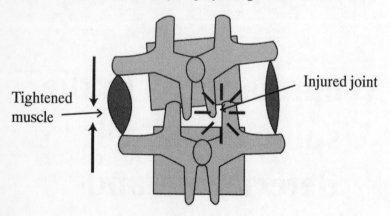

Tightened muscle

Injured joint

Muscles "splint" an injured joint.

---

*   The initial injury is often small or not even noticable. For example, it may be repeated bending and twisting, a childhood fall, or even sleeping with the neck crooked. Chapter eight discusses injury in a lot more detail.

Altered spinal movement

With one joint splinted (and usually a bit crooked), while others move too much, the movement of the spine becomes abnormal. If the injured joint stiffens while it is healing, or the joint is repeatedly injured (for example repeated bending and twisting) this abnormal movement will remain. If uncorrected, the processes described in the rest of this chapter cause damage and deterioration that adds up over years.

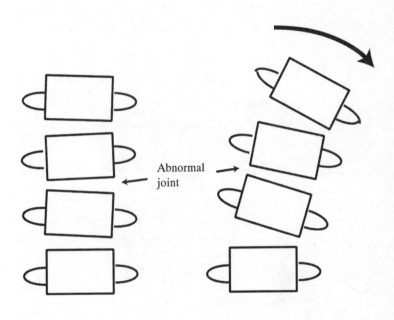

Abnormal joint

When standing the abnormal joint may be a bit crooked.

When trying to bend the abnormal joint makes movement become quite abnormal.

Ongoing damage

Out of balance or forced to move to far, sliding surfaces that normally rub gently may grind forcefully. There will be ongoing damage and the joints will be slightly red and swollen.

Just as mild sunburn is not sore unless slapped, the damaged joints will not be painful unless ground together hard. The body will try to avoid movements that do this.

Out of balance joints rub and grind.

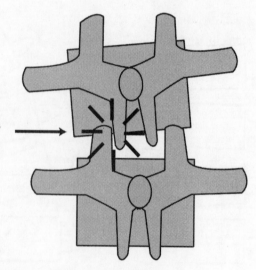

Ongoing damage in an out of balance spine.

Nerve interference

Where the nerves leave the spine they may be irritated or pinched upon. This has very serious consequences, and will be covered in more detail in chapter seven.

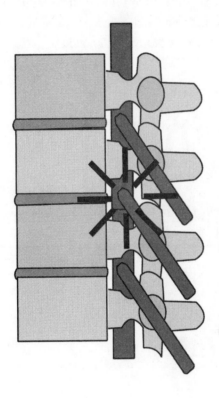

Nerve irritated as it leaves the spine.

Muscular

straining when out of balance

Trying to restore balance, muscles on one side will be constantly pulling. Overworked and unable to rest, they will become tight and tender (sore to touch but not painful). Blood flow will be reduced causing a build up of waste products and a lack of nutrients. A masseur would find the muscles to be "ropy" or "knotted".

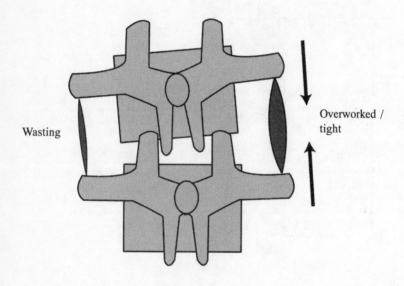

Wasting

Overworked / tight

Joint out of balance. Some muscles are tight and overworked. Others do little and waste away.

Straining to protect the spine from damage

When part of the spine is injured or grinding badly the body will try and protect the spine from damage. One way it does this is to pull tightly with muscles to either take pressure off or to reduce movement.

Muscles may tighten strongly enough to cause obvious muscle spasm.

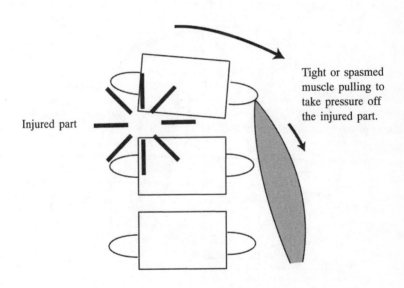

Injured part

Tight or spasmed muscle pulling to take pressure off the injured part.

When part of the spine is injured or damaged, muscles tighten to protect it. This may cause spasm.

Overload elsewhere

When a part of the spine is not doing its normal job, other parts are forced to do extra work. The overloaded parts may become overstressed and damaged.

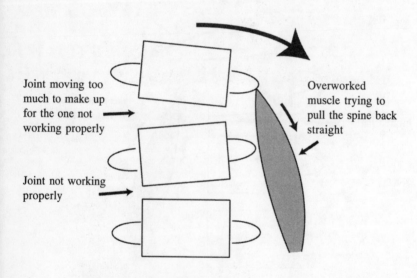

Joint moving too much to make up for the one not working properly →

Overworked muscle trying to pull the spine back straight

Joint not working properly →

A joint not working causes overload elsewhere.

Stiffening and wasting.

The less a stiffened joint is used the weaker it gets. The weaker it gets the less the body will use it. A vicious circle results.

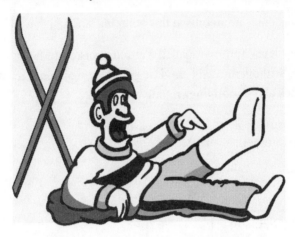

Just as a leg in a cast weakens, so do stiff spinal joints.

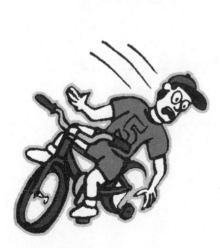

The original injury may be a simple childhood fall.

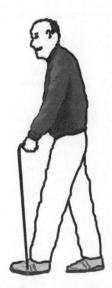

Years later, after the processes of stiffening and weakening.

Starving the discs and joint linings of nutrients

Neither the disc nor the lining of the sliding joints have tiny blood vessels. Regular movement pumps fluid through them like a sponge.

Once a joint becomes immobilised this pumping stops.

Starved of nutrients and overloaded by toxic waste products, the cells may die. Without the cells providing ongoing maintenance and repair, the discs and joint linings rapidly deteriorate.

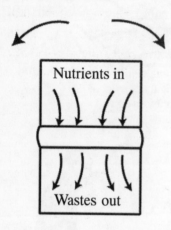

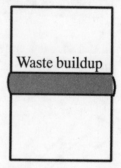

Normal movement pumps nutrients in and wastes out.

No movement. No pumping. Discs and joints are starved of nutrients and build up waste products.

Re-adaptation of ligaments and muscles

Normally ligaments and muscles will be just loose enough to allow normal movement.

Too loose and the joint will slop around. Too tight and the joint will not move freely.

When the movement of a joint changes ligaments and muscles gradually re-adapt. In the example shown the joint has been stuck to the right. The ligaments and muscles have become long on the left and short on the right.

Now changed, the shortened ligaments and muscles will not allow the joint to move to the left. The lengthened ligaments and muscles may be loose enough to allow the joint to slop around and maybe make cracking noises when moving to the right.

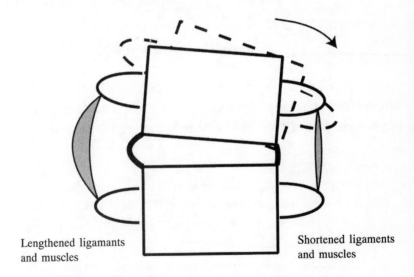

Lengthened ligamants and muscles

Shortened ligaments and muscles

The muscles and ligaments have re-adapted to suit the abnormal movement. The joint cannot move well to the left and moves too far to the right, making cracking noises.

Re-adaptation of bone

As young bone grows it adapts to the stress it is placed under. If a joint is crooked or out of balance for a long time the young bone will grow abnormally. For example, it may grow wedge shaped rather than flat

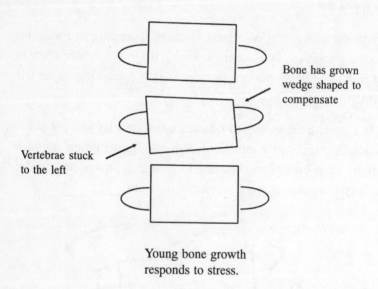

Bone has grown wedge shaped to compensate

Vertebrae stuck to the left

Young bone growth responds to stress.

When an older bone is placed under abnormal stress it will respond by growing spurs of bone. This is the body's attempt to stabilise the area.

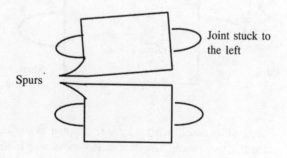

Joint stuck to the left

Spurs

Older bone forms spurs to stabilise joint.

Altered neurological control

What is neurological control?

Try an experiment. Close your eyes and have someone move your finger. Without opening your eyes you will know exactly which direction the finger is pointing. Why?

There are sensors in the muscles and ligaments around every joint. They detect things such as pressure, tightness and length. The brain receives this information and knows what is happening.

Changes in abnormal joints

When the joint movement changes the muscles and ligaments are under abnormal strain and change over time. With these changes muscles and ligaments send inaccurate information to the brain.

Lets see what happens when the brain receives inaccurate information.

Example One

The brain may think that a spinal joint is nicely balanced when it is not. Because of this the spine will be slightly bent or crooked.

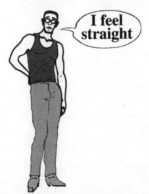

Joint sensors send wrong information.

Example Two

The brain relies on feedback information from the joints to know how far they have moved. Based on the inaccurate information, the body will move too much or too little.

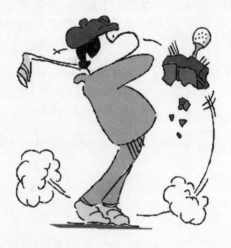

Without correct signals from the joints the brain cannot control movements as well.

Example Three

The brain needs lots of information to balance the body. This information comes from the eyes, the inner ears, and sensors in the joints (especially those of the neck).

With any of this information missing balance and co-ordination are reduced. Try balancing blindfolded. If different pieces of information contradict each other the brain may become confused or dizzy.

For example, spinning around quickly causes the fluid in the inner ear to swish around giving false balance information causing dizziness. Watching a roller coaster or car going around corners on a big screen can give a person motion sickness. Similarly, inaccurate information from the sensors in the spine can cause dizziness, poor balance, and poor co-ordination.

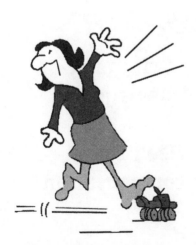

The original injury may be minor.

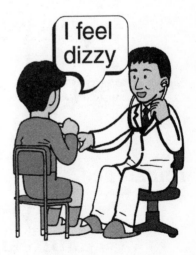

Changes to the way the joints move may cause dizziness years later.

The vicious circle

Once the processes start it becomes a bit like a snowball rolling down a hill. Each aspect tends to make the others worse. For example, a tightening of a small muscle tends to reduce movement and worsen imbalance. This causes:

- stiffness and weakening;

- a reduction of pumping of nutrients to the disc and joint lining;

- an increase in grinding and on-going damage;

- and an increased need for compensation elsewhere.

It gets worse and worse over time without the person knowing. Eventually it may get bad enough to cause pain. This is why pain sometimes starts for no apparent reason.

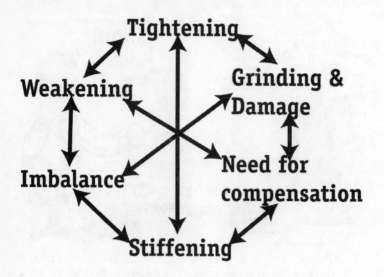

Each part of the problem makes the others worse.

What is this condition called?

What do you call a condition where the spine works abnormally and so many things seem to be affected.

Chiropractors are the fore-runners in the field of diagnosing and treating these complex problems. They call the underlying condition a Vertebral Subluxation Complex, or a "subluxation" for short*. The specialised procedures used to correct a subluxation are called adjustments.

Outside of the chiropractic profession the naming is not so clear.

Why?

Sometimes the complex inter-relationships are not understood. Sometimes practitioners only focus on part of the problem. Sometimes it is easier to tell a patient something simple.

As a result patients can be told all sorts of stories.

---

*   The medical profession have a different meaning for the word "subluxation". This creates confusion sometimes. To make this book clear and easy to read, specialised terms are avoided whenever possible. The term subluxation will be used only sparingly.

"Your muscles and ligaments are out."

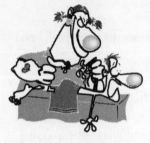

"It's an evil spirit."

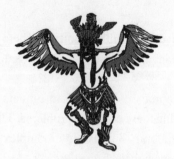

"You've strained it."

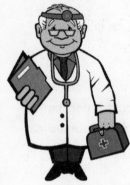

Everyone seems to say something different

"Definately inflamed."

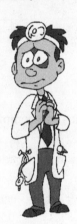

"You have a disc problem."

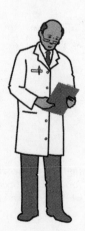

"Your muscles are very tight."

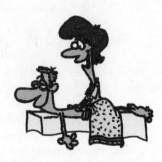

Chapter Three

How spinal problems rob energy, vitality and health

How spinal problems rob energy, vitality and health

Introduction

The problems with the spine and the processes described in the previous chapter rob a person of energy, vitality and health. Here are some of the reasons why.

Ongoing trauma

Anyone who has been in a fight, played contact sport, or done anything that physically knocks themselves around will realise that trauma drains a person.

Make no mistake. Parts that hurt when moved or pressed upon are experiencing trauma. If your x-rays show damage or degeneration you will have suffered trauma. It may not be as obvious as a fall or a blow, but there is trauma in the form of ongoing stress and damage.

Abnormal stress on muscles

Muscles trying to hold a crooked spine straight or trying to protect a spine from damage, work abnormally hard. This takes enormous amounts of energy and is very tiring.

Overcoming stiffened joints

Overcoming stiffness of the joints to move takes a lot of energy and is very tiring.

Inability to rest

Abnormal spines cause muscles to be tight, even when sleeping. This robs the muscles of the rest they need to recover, rebuild and heal..

Interference to the nervous system

Problems with the spine cause interference with the nervous system. This has wide reaching effects on health, as will be discussed in detail in chapter seven.

The effect of pain

Ongoing pain is physically and mentally draining, especially when it interferes with sleep.

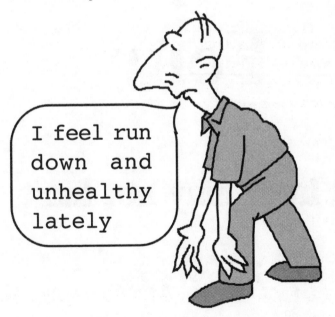

Even if they are not hurting, problems in the spine can rob a person of energy, vitality and health.

Chapter Four

Why it may not hurt for years

Why it may not hurt for years

A tooth may slowly decay for years before irritating a nerve to cause pain. Spines also often "decay" for years (often decades) before becoming sore. Examples such as the following are extremely common.

1.   An older person may walk along bent and crooked, appearing as though there is a "stick up their back-side". Although in a severe condition, they may not feel pain.

2.   Patients go to a clinic with their first experience of back pain, yet X-rays show that one or more of their joints have badly worn. Usually the problem has been there for twenty years or more to cause this damage.

3.   Grown men have felt completely normal, yet their spines are in such bad condition that they bend over to pick up something as light as a pen, and a disc ruptures, sometimes requiring surgery.

In some ways it is most unfortunate that they did not have pain earlier, because most of these conditions are preventable if detected early.

Why can a spine deteriorate so badly, yet not hurt? The following processes show how.

Muscular

Before pain

The muscles that are under abnormal strain will become tight and develop tender "knots". Patients often do not realize that they are sore until someone, such as a masseur, finds them.

Pain eventually occurs because

- something such as a strain, a chill, or extra activity aggravates the tender "knotted muscle";
- the tight muscle tears.

examples
- "muscular" back problems;
- hamstring and groin injuries.

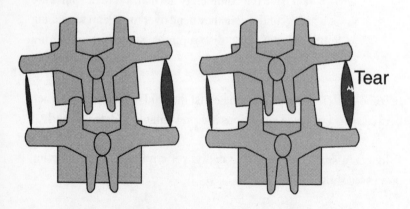

The muscle on the right is under abnormal strain.

Because of this it is easily injured.

Disc Rupture

Before pain

Only the very outside of a disc has nerves that detect damage and send a pain signal to the brain. The inside of a disc can be badly damaged and a person may not feel a thing.

Pain eventually occurs when

- a tear inside a disc has worked from the inside to the outside where the nerves can detect the damage;
- The disc may also bulge outwards and press on a nerve, or rupture completely;
- the discs, which are shock absorbing pads between the vertebrae, rupture leaving a permanent "flat tyre" in the spine.

examples
- someone who feels a pain in the back, then pain that goes down the leg;
- someone who has a series of minor back pains, then has a bad attack that won't go away.

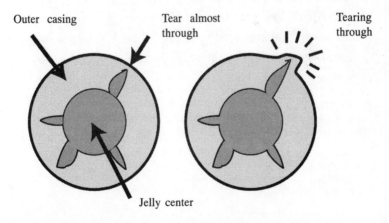

Outer casing

Tear almost through

Tearing through

Jelly center

Tear almost through: no pain.

Tear right through: lots of pain and big trouble!!

Grinding and irritation

Before pain

Spinal joints normally slide gently. When they rub together a bit harder they become mildly swollen. Just as mild sunburn is not sore until touched, the mildly swollen joints will not be painful unless they rub a bit harder.

The body realises which activities and movements cause the joints to rub together harder. These are avoided where possible.

Eventually pain occurs because

- the damage caused by the rubbing becomes severe;
- the spine becomes a bit more crooked or so out of balance that the rubbing or grinding gets worse;
- certain activities or movements increase the rubbing and grinding.

Examples

- a sore back that gradually gets worse over the years (damage accumulates and imbalances get worse);
- a sore back that goes away with rest and gets sore when the person "does something stupid" (there is mild grinding that flares up with certain activities and movements, then settles down when rested).

Before pain

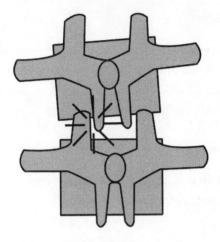

Moderate rubbing - no pain.

Pain

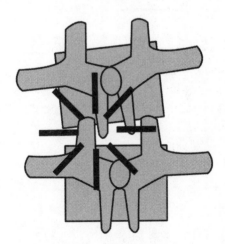

Hard grinding - eventual pain.

Irritation to a nerve

Before pain

The holes the nerves leave the spine through are normally large enough to allow plenty of room for the nerves. As the spine becomes worn or unbalanced the hole may become smaller. Scar tissue, swelling or disc bulges may reduce the size of the hole still further.

Pain eventually occurs because

- the swelling, scar tissue, or other parts move that final millimeter to actually touch the nerve.

Examples
- sciatica (leg pain);
- numbness, tingling or weakness in the arm or hand;
- headache.

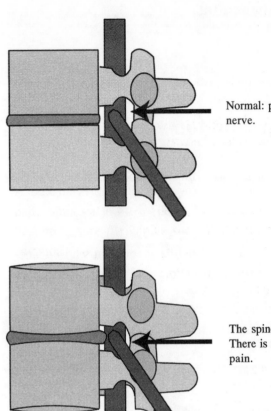

Normal: plenty of room for the nerve.

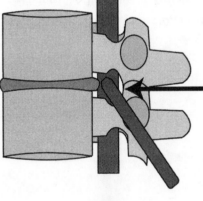

The spine has deteriorated. There is a lot less room: but no pain.

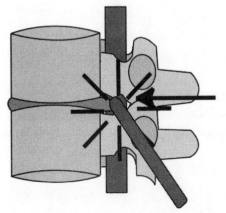

The spine has deteriorated further, starting to press on the nerve causing pain.

Failure due to weakening

Before pain

Like an arm that has become weak in a sling, a weak spinal joint will not hurt.

Eventually pain occurs because

- the joint becomes so weak that parts become damaged with use.

Example
- a person whose back had not been sore, but whose spine had weakened gradually over time, then when bent over had his or her back go "twang".

Seizing up

Before pain

The spine gets gradually stiffer and stiffer. A person will subconsciously compensate by moving less, often becoming noticably stiffer as they get older.

Pain eventually results from

- the spine becoming too stiff to do normal movements;
- the spine becoming seized completely.

examples

- people who to have a stiff or crooked spine. When doing things within their limitations they are OK. When they try to do a bit more (something a person with a reasonably healthy spine would do easily) their spine gives trouble.

Overloading other parts

Before pain

Part of the spine is not working normally, forcing other parts such as joints, muscles or ligaments to do work they were not meant to. This is called *compensating*. There is no pain when the overworked parts are coping with the extra work.

The body subconsciously understands that there is a problem, and avoids activities and movements that increase the strain on these overworked parts.

Pain eventually occurs because

•   the compensating parts strain, are damaged, or can no longer cope with the extra workload.

Compensations are extremely common!
The majority of people with spinal problems have some sort of pain due to compensations.

Note: Sometimes this is referred to as the cart horse phenomena. If two horses are pulling a cart, and one stops pulling, eventually the good horse gets sore or starts to complain. In the case of the cart horses it may be obvious where the problem is. In the spine it may not be obvious. Many practitioners only give some feel good type of treatment to the sore spots without finding the real cause. It is a bit like giving the overworked good cart horse a rest, a nice rub down and a few sugar cubes. It will be happy for a while, but will eventually get sore and complain again, or worse still, break down completely.

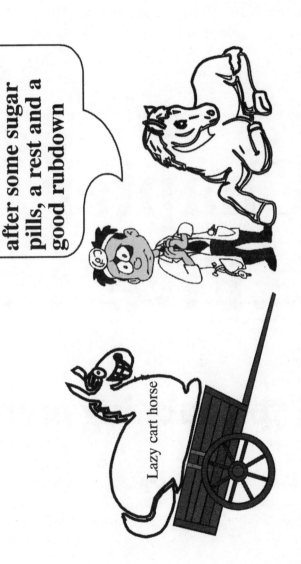

If one part of the spine does not work, another may get sore.

Chapter Five

Are you painting over rust?

Are you painting over rust?

Every day in clinics around the world a scene is acted out. A patient will walk in with a sore back. The practitioner does something that is believed to fix the problem. The patient feels better for a while. Sometimes the practitioner's charisma or sales pitch is so good, or the pain relief so dramatic, that the practitioner is seen to be almost some sort of magical guru.

Most people knowledgable about back problems understand that there is a second part to this story. Eventually the problem returns and needs fixing again. As the years go by it needs to be fixed more often. The problem gets a bit worse, and often becomes harder to fix. Often the patient will eventually become desperate or frustrated and look for a new magical guru.

What happens? Does the magical guru lose all his or her magic?

The truth is that there was never any magic in the first place. The guru's fixes are often no more impressive than painting over a rust bucket car and claiming to have repaired the damage. Eventually the rust bubbles through the paint. Underneath, the panels continue to deteriorate. Unfortunately "rust" in a spine is not so visible, and may take 20 years to show through badly.

What actually happens

Most problems in the spine originate from injuries that cause the spine to work abnormally. Working abnormally, parts of the spine rub, grind, or are placed under abnormal stress. Pain occurs when one of these parts eventually "gives out".

Often the magical gurus merely patch up the part that gives out, appearing to have fixed the problem. Despite impressive claims, rarely are the underlying problems fixed.

How to pick 'painting over rust' treatments

The remainder of this chapter describes some common 'painting over rust' treatments. Common characteristics include:
- they promise some sort of 'fix' in a short amount of time, and
- they are often simplistic.

These approaches should be compared with a more realistic plan that actually address the underlying problems. One such plan is presented in chapter eleven.

Putting a bone back in

The belief

A manipulator puts a bone back in place.

What actually happens

Many excellent practitioners make 'popping' noises in the spine to help restore normal movement and balance. These procedures are called adjustments, and can form part of genuine quality care.

Many popping noises unfortunately are caused by crude procedures that temporarily free up the spine. The popping noise is the sound of stuck surfaces separating.

Temporarily the spine may feel better. Things are moving and some pressure has come off the muscles, nerves and ligaments, but eventually the spine will return to the way it was. The joint will re-seize, become overloaded, or be damaged again.

Why?

The problem joint will have stiffened or deteriorated. Muscles and ligaments will have shortened, weakened, or otherwise changed. The joint will no longer be capable of doing its normal job, and the body will have made adaptations to have other joints do the work.

Chapter twelve explains how to tell the difference between 'pops' that give only temporary relief, and 'pops' which form part of quality care that produces long term benefit.

Massage and 'muscle manipulation'

The belief

"It's a muscular problem", or "there is a muscle out that needs to be put back in".

What actually happens

Muscles usually tighten because of imbalances in the spine, irritation to a nerve, or to protect a damaged part. Massage will relieve the painful muscles, but with the underlying cause remaining, the muscles will re-tighten.

More forceful masseurs sometimes call themselves muscle manipulators. They find tight bands of muscle which they interpret as a muscle out of place.

Muscles are firmly attached at each end and enclosed in very strong sheaths, so they cannot go "out". After giving the tight muscle a firm flick it temporarily relaxes. Not feeling a tight band of muscle afterwards, the muscle manipulators wrongly believe that they have put the muscle back where it belongs.

Of course the muscles will re-tighten, seeming to require regular "putting back".

Before massage or 'muscle manipulation'

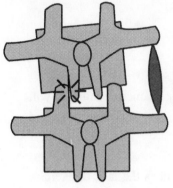

Tightened muscle

The muscle is tightened trying to balance or protect the spine.

After massage or 'muscle manipulation'

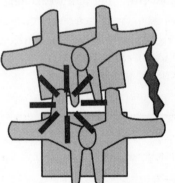

Temporarily loosened muscle

Later

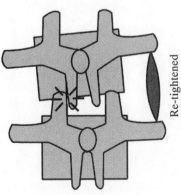

Re-tightened muscle

The muscle has temporarily loosened. Imbalances and grinding may increase without protection from the muscle.

The muscle has re-tightened.

Rest

The belief

Rest and it gets better.

What really happens

Of course any part that is being abnormally strained or damaged will feel better if rested. When one stops resting the abnormal strain and damage will continue.

When a spine rests for more than a few days the lack of exercise causes more stiffening and weakening. The underlying problems actually worsen. Prolonged rest is recognised now as an inappropriate and very damaging form of spinal treatment.

Magic rubs and sprays

The belief

Rubbing or spraying something on the injury fixes the problem.

What actually happens

There are two basic versions.

1. The so called heat rubs. Putting heat on an injury is actually dangerous (see p.100). Luckily the heat rubs do not really heat things much. They actually irritate the skin making a hot sensation, which blocks pain by a simple neurological trick. The irritation messages from the skin block the pain messages from getting through.

    It works the same way that rubbing a sore spot sometimes lessens pain.

2. The cold sprays act like ice, numbing the area.

Ligament and tendon manipulation

The belief

Ligaments and tendons are put back in place to help re-align and hold the bones in.

What really happens

Ligaments are the hard white fibrous tissue that is found around a joint, such as those found in a leg of lamb. Like the muscles they are firmly attached and cannot go "out".

Tendons are the smooth, round, rope-like structures that attach muscles to bone. They are usually firmly encased in a sheath, and unless a significant rupture occurs, they cannot deviate from their course either.

When injured, a tendon or ligament will often become bound or irritated by scar tissue. Manipulation or firm rubbing often frees tendons or ligaments. If the pain is coming from the tendons or ligaments, pain may be reduced dramatically.

Many educated practitioners use forms of treatment that break up bindings and scar tissue. A common one is called friction massage. Although very useful, bound or irritated ligaments and tendons are usually only part of an overall complex problem.

Analgesics and anti inflammatory drugs

The belief

Take these tablets. They will fix it.

What actually happens

Anti-inflammatory drugs
Inflammation is the body's natural healing response to damage. Part of this response includes the production of a pain signal to warn the brain of the damage so as further injury can be prevented. Anti-inflammatory drugs stop inflammation, thereby stopping pain.

Analgesics
Analgesics block pain signals from getting to the brain.

The danger

Without pain as a warning, the body will not know to avoid damaging movements and activities. The situation is like cutting the wire to a flashing dashboard temperature light and continuing to drive, believing that the overheating problem has been fixed.

Some examples of other things that can relieve pain, making people feel better when they are not.
• Some applications of electrical devices (eg. T.E.N.S., interferential).
• Some applications of acupuncture.
• Some sprays and rubs.
• Some applications of ultrasound.

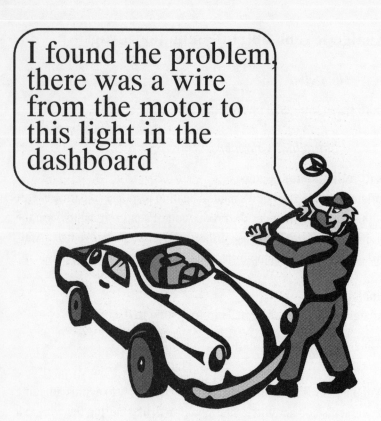

Though it would be clearly stupid to disconnect a flashing warning light in a car's dashboard, many forms of treatment for back pain stop pain from registering in the brain while leaving the actual problem uncorrected.

Exercise

The belief

Stretching and / or strengthening will fix a bad back.

What actually happens

There are many ways stretching or strengthening alone may relieve
back problems. In general they can be likened to sending the good
but worn out cart horse (see page 46) to the gym. It will make the
compensating parts better able to cope, but may do nothing to fix the
real problems. The exercising alone usually worsen imbalances and
make the joints work more abnormally.

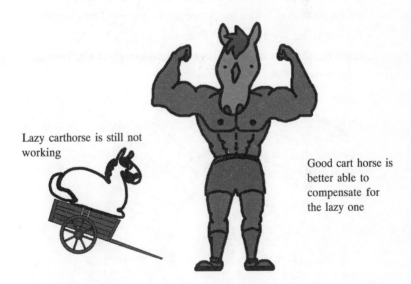

Lazy carthorse is still not
working

Good cart horse is
better able to
compensate for
the lazy one

Exercising alone when the spine is not working properly just
improves the compensating part's ability to compensate.

The technical stuff

- Where a muscle is tight, stretching will relieve the tightness and soreness. The muscles will re-tighten because the underlying imbalance, nerve interference or damage remain.

- Exercises designed to increase the movement of the spine will make the spine bend more, but only the joints that are free will stretch. The stuck joints will stay stuck. Instead of uniform movement, the compensating free joints will become loose and sloppy, while the stiff joints remain stiff. The sloppy joints may become so unstable that they start to make popping noises and movement causes damage. Sloppy joints are extremely difficult, if not impossible to restore to normal.

- Exercise can strengthen the muscles that are attempting to balance an out of balance joint, or joints that are compensating for ones that won't work. Sure the spine is better able to cope, but the very abnormal mechanical system is reinforced, not removed.

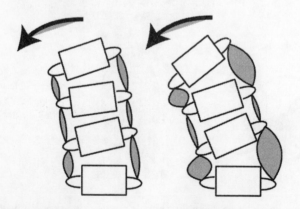

Before exercise
Middle joint not moving. Others are compensating.

After exercise
Middle joint still stiff and weak. Compensating joints moving too much. Their muscles well developed.

Chapter Six

X-ray changes

How deterioration is seen on X-rays.

Normal

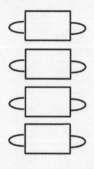 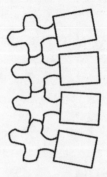

From the front all the bones should look as though they are sitting balanced on top of each other.

From the side the bones should form a smooth curve with equal spaces between them.

Mainly muscle and ligament damage plus some disc deformation (sometimes called phase1)

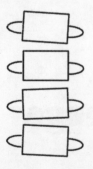 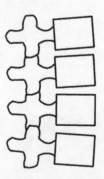

From the front some bones may look as though they are sitting crooked. The discs have become wedge shaped. The muscles and ligaments have deteriorated.

From the side the curve is not smooth, and may have straightened. Again this shows changes in the muscles, ligaments and discs.

Deterioration of the bones and discs, plus gross changes to the muscles and ligaments. (phase 2)

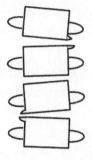
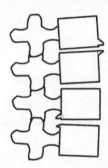

From the front the bones may sit crooked. Spurs of bone may be seen growing out the side.

From the side some of the spaces between the bones are smaller, showing that the disc between the bones has broken down. There may be spurs of bone.

Gross degeneration (phase 3)

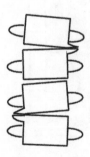
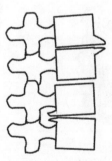

From the front, large spurs of bone may be seen. Bones may be very crooked.

From the side the spaces between the bones may be very small or have disappeared. Some discs have broken down. Large spurs of bone are seen.

Can X-rays find problems in the spine

Imagine driving a car and hitting a big pot hole. The wheels become out of alignment and out of balance. The car shudders and wanders. The tyres start to wear rapidly and unevenly.

It would be little use checking the tyres straight away to find out why the car shudders and wanders. They will not show bad wear patterns until maybe 10- 20,000 km later.

Taking X-rays of a spine is often like checking the tyre wear to find why a car shudders and wanders[#]. X-rays usually only show the damage that occurs secondary to the underlying problem.[*] However, this damage may eventually become a significant problem in its own right.

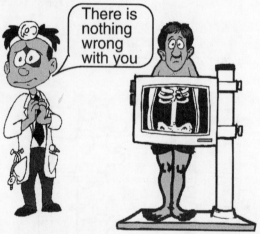

Wrong! X-rays often do not show the primary problem, only the secondary damage caused after many years*

[#]   X-rays are often needed to look for problems such as tumours, fractures, certain diseases, and other problems.

[*]   This is true for most professionals, however some practitioners such as chiropractors are trained to look for evidence of imbalance and abnormal mechanics as well.

Is degeneration or "arthritis" a consequence of old age?

After 20,000 km the owner of the car that hit the pot hole notices bad wear on the left front tyre. The other tyres are near new. Only a complete fool would suggest that the tyre was worn because of "old age".

On the other hand, a patient's X-ray will show one or a few badly worn spinal joints, while the rest are completely normal, yet some professionals unfortunately blame the worn joints on "old age".

The truth usually is that the worn joints have been out of adjustment and wearing abnormally for many years. Rather than being a natural expectation, they are the result of a problem that most probably could have been fixed or prevented.

Avoiding "arthritis"

A sensible way of avoiding arthritis in old age is to :
- exercise regularly;
- avoid damaging activities (see chapter eight);
- have your spine regularly checked by a person skilled in examining and adjusting the spine. He or she will find and correct the abnormalities that cause accellerated wear and deterioration; and,
- eat a healthy diet.

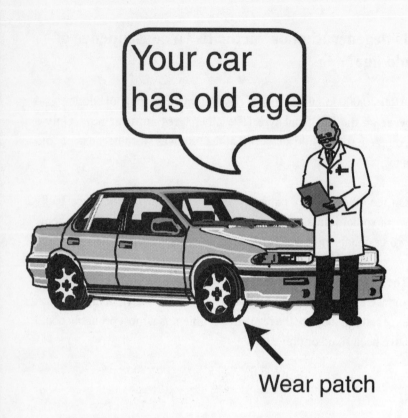

Wear patch

Although this is obviously stupid, the same thing happens with spines every day!

Chapter Seven

Nerve interference

Interference to the nerves

What are nerves?

Nerves are the electrical wiring that the brain uses to send and receive messages.

Why is interference to nerves a concern?

Interference to the nerves cause things such as sciatica, numbness and tingling in the hands and fingers, and headaches. However, over the past 100 years chiropractors have noticed that seemingly unrelated problems appeared to be cured following adjustments to the spine. These problems include conditions such as indigestion, period pain, asthma, bed wetting, and ear infections.

How does this happen?

Science now understands that if a nerve is irritated one of two things will happen. Sometimes the signals are blocked or partially blocked. Other times the irritation causes extra signals like static on a telephone line.

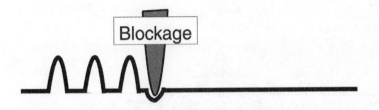

Normal nerve flow   Nerve flow after blockage

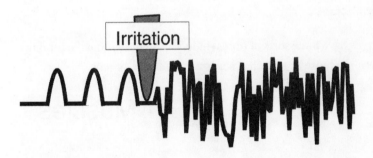

Normal nerve flow   Nerve flow after irritation

To understand how this effects the body lets look at where the nerves go and what sort of messages are sent through them. Nerves pass from the spinal cord to almost everywhere in the body as shown.

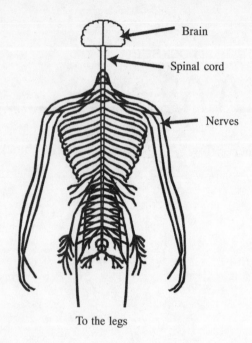

To the legs

Nerves have three sorts of fibres (individual wires within the cabling). These are those to muscles, sensory, and to the organs.

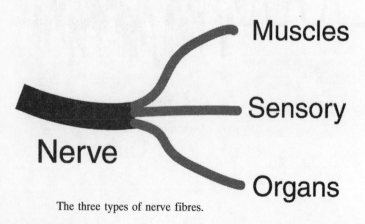

The three types of nerve fibres.

Nerves to muscles

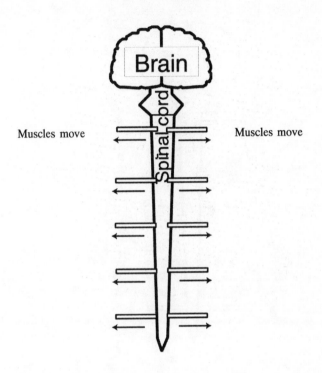

What happens when nerves to muscles are irritated

Blockages cause muscles to weaken. Static causes muscles to tighten or spasm.

Sensory nerves

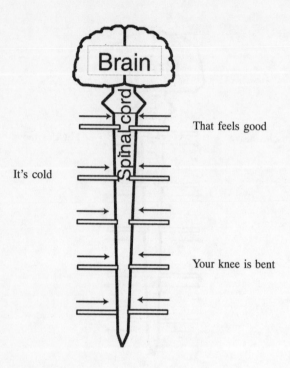

What happens when sensory fibres are irritated

Blockage causes numbness or a loss of feeling altogether. Static causes pain such as sciatica and headaches.

Irritation to the sensory nerves also cause the brain to receive inaccurate information from the joints of the body. As discussed on pages 27-29 if the brain receives the inaccurate information there can be postural changes, poor coordination, dizziness and poor balance.

Nerves to the organs

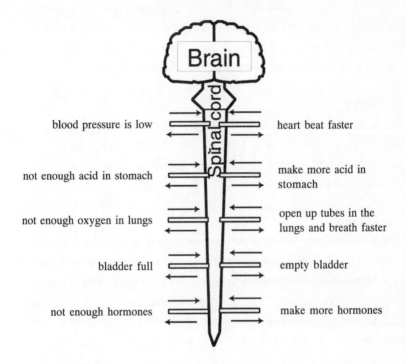

What happens when nerves to the organs are irritated

If the nerves to the organs are irritated almost anything can happen. Lets look at some possible examples.

The stomach

Heart burn or ulcers are caused by too much acid. Just as too much acid can be produced in so called "nervous stomachs", it may be produced if the nerves to the stomach get a lot of static. The same thing may occur if the signal telling the brain how much acid is in the stomach is blocked. If the brain wrongly thinks there is not enough acid it will tell the stomach to make more.

The heart
If someone has a fright the brain will tell the heart to beat faster. If the nerve to the heart has static the heart may beat faster too, causing high blood pressure. The same thing may occur if the signal telling the brain about the blood pressure is blocked. The brain may wrongly think the blood pressure is too low and tell the heart to beat faster.

The lungs
When some people get scared they get so called nervous asthma. Their brain sends out a signal and the tubes in the lungs tighten. The same thing may happen if there is irritation causing static to the nerves to the lungs.

The bladder
When the bladder is full a message is sent to the bladder control centre. The bladder control centre does routine things, but receives general instructions from the brain. In a very young person whenever the bladder control centre gets the message that the bladder is full, a message is automatically sent to empty it. After a while the brain learns to control this, firstly while awake, then when asleep.

Of course, if the bladder is really, really, full the nerve signals will be so strong that the bladder control centre will basically say to the brain "I'm going to empty the bladder no matter what you say!!!"

Static in a younger person may make the signals so strong that the brain cannot control things when asleep. Bedwetting may result.

In an older person with a very bad spine the static may be so strong that the brain cannot control things at all.

Medical opinion on nerve interference as a cause of these problems

Medical practitioners well recognise nerve interference as a cause of both sciatica, and numbness and tingling in the hands and fingers. Most are beginning to recognise interference in the neck as being a cause of headaches.

Although the same neurological principles apply, the standard medical line is that nerve interference from the spine does not cause the problems described previously, or any other seemingly un-related disease. Patients with these conditions are unlikely to have their spines checked. Funds are unlikely to be allocated to research the issue. The scientific principles behind nerve interference causing disease are not likely to figure prominently in medical education and literature.

Why? The most probable reasons are purely related to economics and to the protection of professional 'territories'. Simply, if everyone had their spines checked regularly, and by removing nerve interference they remained much healthier or recovered from disease better, there would be much less need for drugs and other medical services.

Special message

Spinal nerve irritation is only one cause of disease. Chiropractors certainly do not claim to be able to cure all disease by correcting the spine. It is up to the qualified practitioner/chiropractor to tell what is the cause and appropriate care in each case.

Chapter Eight

How a spine is injured

How a spine is injured

Most of the damage to a spine happens during the years and decades after an initial injury. This happens through the processes described in chapter two. What causes the initial injury though?

Injury

There are three common ways a spine can be injured: once off trauma, repeated trauma, and prolonged strain.

Once off trauma

This is self explanatory. A spine can be injured by any significant trauma. It may range from a motor vehicle accident or sporting injury through to having one's head pulled and twisted when being born.

Repeated trauma

If parts of the spine are repeatedly overstressed they can gradually break down or become inflamed. By far the most common repeated overstresses are i), unsafe lifting and ii), bending and twisting. Both of these place tremendous leverage on the lower back.

To understand lifting one must understand the basic principles of leverage.

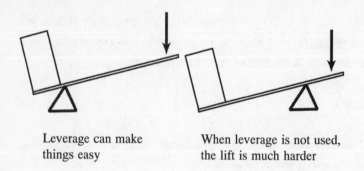

Leverage can make things easy

When leverage is not used, the lift is much harder

Lets see how the principles of leverage work with lifting.

When a person lifts, the fulcrum (leverage point) is at the base of the spine. When the load is close to the body the leverage is favorable. When bent over, the load is a long way from the fulcrum. Leverage multiplies this weight by about ten times. If the load is 10 kg, the load on the spine is about 100 kg.

Safe lift   **Unsafe lift**

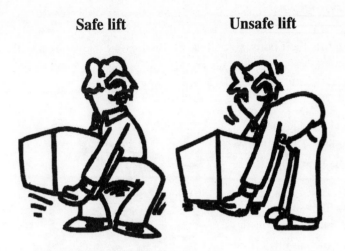

Load close to body and
leverage point.

Spine vertical

Load a long way
from leverage
point.

Spine more horizintal

Fulcrum (leverage
point)

Fulcrum
(leverage
point)

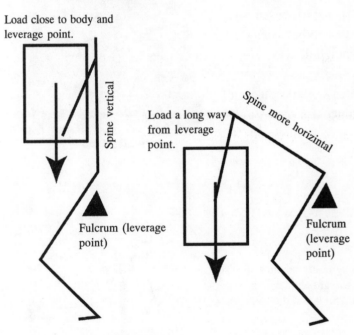

Body weight

A person lifts their body as well as the load. An 80 kg person will have about 50 kg above their waist (the trunk, arms, neck and head). When bent over, leverage on the spine will be about five times.

With this leverage the 50 kg body weight adds 250 kg load to the bent spine.

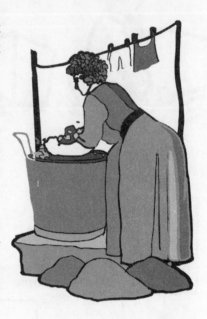

As an example, a housewife hanging out clothes on the line may put about 250kg load on her back each bend, even though the clothing only weighs a little.

If there are 100 pieces of clothing that means a 250 kg load is incurred 100 times.

Although only bending over, the body weight and leverage puts about 250 kg on the spine.

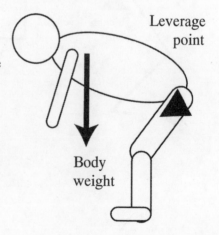

Leverage point

Body weight

Comparison of lifting techniques

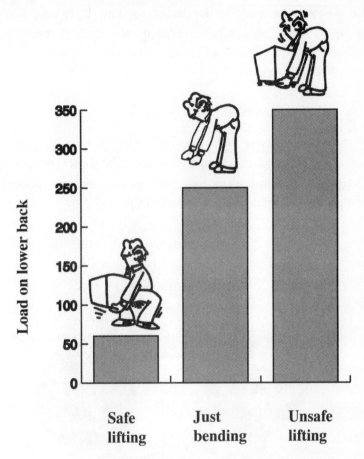

Because the body's weight is lifted there is a lot more strain on the back lifting a feather unsafely than there is lifting a moderate load safely.

Experience from the real world

Manual handling consultancy for industry shows that people usually make a reasonable try at lifting heavy things safely, but are very careless and do a lot of damage lifting lighter things.

Bending and twisting

Lower backs are really not designed to twist much, Twists put a lot
of strain on the parts. When combined with bending, stresses are
enormous. Often someone will bend and twist then a disc badly tears.
This is a major problem.

Prolonged strain

Parts of the spine such as the muscles and ligaments are designed to
do work, relax and recover, then do some more work. They are not
designed to take strain all the time. Some postures and work positions
put parts of the spine under constant strain.

Try this experiment. Put a bowling ball on a short stick. Hold the
stick with the ball balanced, then with it unbalanced (as shown in the
diagram). Balanced is easy, but unbalanced is hard soon tiring the
wrist and hand.

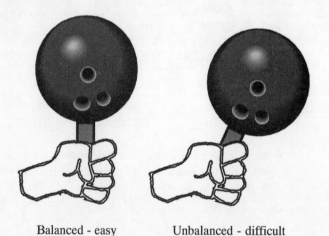

Balanced - easy   Unbalanced - difficult

A head weighs as much as a bowling ball and the neck is about as long as the stick. Having the head forward unbalanced puts a lot of strain on the neck.

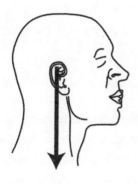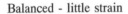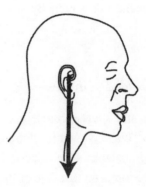

Balanced - little strain   Unbalanced - lots of strain

Another common source of prolonged strain is poor sleeping posture. The following diagram shows a head on a well supporting pillow, and secondly pillow that puts the neck in a bent position. The bent position stretches things on one side of the neck, while jamming things up on the other side.

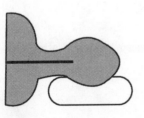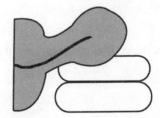

Well supported.   Spine not well supported - lots of strain.

Other things that cause a spine to lock up or move abnormally

Stress

When someone is emotionally stressed or worried often the neck muscles will tighten. Sometimes this can cause joints of the neck to lock up.

One sided activities

Many jobs and sports require each side of the body to be used differently. This may overdevelop muscles on one side of the spine causing an imbalance. One sided activities may also place abnormal strain on the joints on that side of the body.

Special mention: having a baby

When pregnant, there is a lot of extra load on the spine and the big tummy pulls the spine and pelvis forward at a stressful angle. At the same time hormones loosen up ligaments so the pelvis can open up a bit more to allow the baby to pass through.

The birth process can be very stressful on the spine and pelvis, then afterwards the mum in a weakened state has to take care of a new baby. It is no wonder that many cases of spinal problems can be traced back to having babies.

Spinal care is most important during pregnancy and after birth.

It's much worse when the spine is out of balance or not moving normally.

All the things described so far can injure a perfectly healthy spine. If a spine is already out of balance, rubbing and grinding, or overstressing where it shouldn't be, the same things will do a lot of damage.

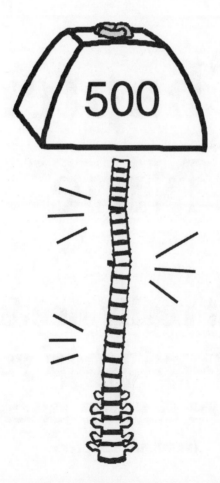

If a spine is already working abnormally
extra load can do a lot of damage.

Chapter Nine

What really needs to be fixed when you have a sore back

(summary chapter)

What really needs to be fixed when you have a sore back

Why a person gets back pain

Usually an injury or something upsets the balance and movement of the spine. This places abnormal stress and load on some parts. Eventually an overloaded or overstressed part 'gives out'. There may be muscle damage, inflammation, pressure on a nerve, a damaged disc, or many other things.

Fix the part that gives out, or fix the cause?

The 'paint over rust' treatments described in chapter five typically only help to 'fix' the parts that give out, or worse, block the pain so the brain is not aware of the problem.

If a practioner does a thorough examination he or she will probably find a lot of other parts that are stiff, painful to touch, or not working properly.

Why is this?

Over the years a person will have done many things that may upset the balance and movement of the spine, causing the conditions described above. Chiropractors call these conditions Vertebral Subluxation Complexes or simply 'subluxations'.

Despite the damage they cause and their detrimental effects to health and wellbeing, subluxations may not cause pain until something gives out. This may take many years (or decades). Without pain as a warning, a spine can accumulate many subluxations.

Quality lasting care of the spine must not only address the part that 'gives' out, but also the underlying subluxation complexes.

What must be done to correct a subluxation complex

After only six weeks in a cast, a broken arm changes dramatically. Muscles waste away and the joint becomes stiff.

By the time subluxation complexes become painful, the changes to the spine are usually much more significant.

Some important changes

Changes to the ligamants
Where the spine has restricted movement the ligaments will quickly shorten. These shortened ligamants will then prevent full movement.

Where the spine is forced to move too much the ligamants will stretch and lengthen over time. The lengthened ligaments will then allow the spine to move too much, often resulting in popping noises.

Changes to muscles

Just as the muscles in an immobilised broken arm deteriorate quickly, so do the muscles in a subluxation complex. They may effect the way the spine works, and become a source of pain in their own right.

The following examples show what often happens.

Weakening or wasting

Spine tilting towards the
opposite side

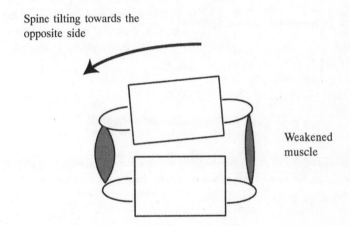

Weakened
muscle

When a muscle weakens or wastes it cannot support its side of the spine, so the spine will tend to tilt towards the opposite side.

Shortening or tightening

When a muscle shortens or tightens the opposite happens. The spine will be pulled towards the same side.

Quite often weakening or tightening of muscles is caused by irritation of the nerve to the muscle. Blockage will cause weakening. Static will cause tightening.

Fibrosis or scar tissue

Fibrosis is like the stringy bits in a poor cut of meat. It can form like scar tissue when the muscle is under prolonged stress, or when it is not being used enough. It stops the muscle shortening and lengthening as it is supposed to. Scar tissue can also form after injury. Sometimes the scar tissue can stick things together.

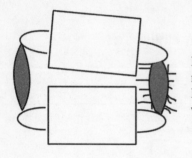

Fibrosis and scar tissue stiffen muscles and stick things together. In this case the scar and fibrosis would stop movement to the left.

Trigger points and other sore spots

Muscles under abnormal stress will develop tight tender spots. Tender means that they are sore when touched. Some of these spots shoot pain to other parts of the body.

When a masseur examines muscles they usually find a lot of sore spots the patient did not know existed. If not found by a practitioner, they often stay un-noticed until something strains or aggravates the muscle.

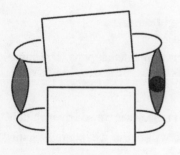

Abnormally stressed muscles develop tender spots which may become sore if aggravated.

Changes to the disc

Discs should be flat shock absorbing pads between the bones. If effected by a subluxation, a disc will deteriorate, possibly becoming thin, stiff, or even wedged shaped.

Disc like this may cause the spine to sit crookedly, or not be able to move freely.

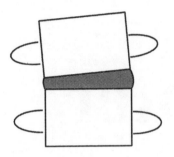

The disc has deteriorated on the left and become wedge shaped. Because of this the spine will sit crooked and not be able to bend freely to the right.

Changes to the shape of bones

Long term the bones in a younger person may grow to be wedge shaped. In an older person the bones may grow 'arthritic' spurs. This is discussed on page 26.

Altered neurological control

After a short period of time the abnormal joints send wrong information about movement and position back to the brain. The brain then thinks that abnormal movement and positions are normal. This is discussed on pages 27-29.

Changes to the way the body does things

The body will also change the way it does things to avoid the movements and activities that damage the abnormal spine. For example it may turn the whole body rather than the neck. These changes become habits that must also be broken.

Chapter Ten

The solution

The Solution

Waiting for pain, then covering up symptoms or doing a patch up does not work. There is a far better way.

The following chapter describes a far superior approach that is used by many wellness oriented chiropractors and some other practitioners. It is logical and works with nature to correct the underlying problem and bring about long term changes. If you have a problem, you should seek out a practitioner who uses this approach.

Whilst remarkable recoveries are sometimes achieved, there is a far better option than having your damaged spine 'fixed'.

The principles that these practitioners use to help an unhealthy spine recover should be part of a healthy lifestyle that prevents problems and enhances life.

There is great wisdom in this.

To summarise the earlier chapters, when a spine is working abnormally many detrimental processes happen. Chiropractors call this a Vertebral Subluxation Complex or simply a subluxation.

Subluxations may eventually cause pain, sickness and other symptoms, but even before these become noticable more sinister changes happen underneath.

Serious 'hidden' consequences of subluxations include degeneration, interference to the nervous system, the placing of abnormal stress on the spine, and the placing of abnormal stress on the body. These can seriously effect health, wellbeing and human potential.

Benefits of a wellness approach

A good wellness oriented chiropractor will use the principles described in the next chapter to help remove subluxations and then help to keep the body subluxation free. Lets look at the human benefits.

Degeneration

X/rays of 80 year old spines often show that some parts are badly worn, yet others are like new. The worn parts were affected by subluxations for years. The un-worn parts were not as affected.

Having a good wellness oriented chiropractor take care of your spine on a regular basis may slow or stop abnormal degeneration. Imagine the 80 year old's life with badly degenerated parts in his or her spine, then imagine the difference in quality of life the wellness approach over the person's lifetime would have made.

Nerve interference

The body has an inbuilt ability to stay healthy and repair itself. The brain controls and coordinates this. Subluxations interfere with this ability by distorting messages sent and received through the nervous system. With subluxations removed this wonderful control system can work freely. Imagine the difference this makes to health and wellbeing.

Abnormal stress on the body

Subluxations place a lot of extra stress on the body. As discussed in chapter three, this drains energy, vitality and health. Imagine the difference to life being subluxation free and regaining that energy and vitality would make.

Abnormal strain on the spine

Subluxations cause abnormal strain on the spine. This makes serious damage much more likely. If spines were kept subluxation free there would be dramatically fewer disc injuries and other debilitating back conditions.

The overall effect

Typically a patient will come to a wellness chiropractor's clinic in pain. Looking beyond the pain, he or she is often run down. Their postures and facial expressions suggest that the weight of the world is on their shoulders. There are often other health problems too.

After patient's subluxations are removed a remarkable change often occurs. It is almost as though the weight is lifted from their shoulders. The patient's facial expressions and posture will change. They will have more energy. They will be getting along better with their families and others. Their health and wellbeing will improve.

The transformation is often so wonderful that we almost forget that the pain goes too.

A wellness chiropractor's clinic can be a remarkable place. Rather than being full of sick and sore people, many will be healthy and feeling great. They view spinal care as a way to enhance health, just like a good diet and regular exercise.

> How different would life be if I took care of my spine when I was younger!

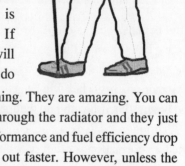

Limp home mode

Some modern cars with electronic management systems have what is called a "limp home mode". If something malfunctions the motor will slow down, do things differently, or do whatever it takes to still keep running. They are amazing. You can pull bits off, and even put an axe through the radiator and they just keep chugging along. Of course performance and fuel efficiency drop off, and the motor probably wears out faster. However, unless the warning lights alert the driver he or she may not even realise!

"Limp home modes" are not new. Humans have always had it. You can pull out a lung and kidney, chop off a leg, clog the arteries with gunk, and the body still keeps chugging along.

From the time you have your neck twisted being born, or fall out of a high chair your spine may be in limp home mode. As one gets older and accumulates more problems the changes limp home mode makes will become more obvious.

Wellness care is not about waiting until a spine finally breaks down, rather it is about keeping the spine and body working the way it was meant to, at optimum performance and efficiency.

Chapter Eleven

The basic three step treatment process

A sensible three step approach

To give lasting benefit, a plan of care must do two things.
*   The parts that are damaged or sore must be helped.
*   The underlying changes must be corrected.
This was discussed in chaper nine.

The following three step approach is sensible and logical for most people.

Step One: Reducion of damage and swelling

Step Two: Restoration and rehabilitation

Step Three: Maintenance

Step one: reduction of damage and swelling

The first thing to do is to relieve the patients symptoms. This is done by reducing damage and swelling. The following treatments may be useful.

Special note: Although many of these treatments are inadequate for making lasting corrections to the spine, as discussed in chapter five, they may be quite useful for reducing damage and swelling.

Rest
Rest takes the load off damaged and swollen parts, allowing nature to take its course and heal. Rest is often wise for a few days, but prolonged rest will cause stiffening and weakening which is very detrimental to the spine.

Ice
If pain is sharp or severe, especially on some movements, there is usually a lot of inflammation (redness and swelling) and maybe some internal bleeding. Ice put on the sore area will reduce inflammation and internal bleeding. Commercial ice packs, crushed ice, and bags of frozen peas all work well. As a guide, they should be applied ten minutes per hour for about 48 hours.

Adjustments
An adjustment is a highly skilled accurate procedure to restore normal movement. Pressure can be taken off damaged parts, muscle spasm reduced, and blood flow increased.

Acupuncture
Acupuncture acts to relieve pain and can stimulate healing.

Massage
Massage may relax painful muscle tightness, allowing increased movement and increased blood flow.

Ultrasound
Ultrasound can reduce pain, reduce swelling and muscle spasm, plus increase blood flow and healing.

Electrical Stimulators
Electrical machines such a T.E.N.S. and Interferential give high frequency (fast) tingling. This acts as an electrical nerve block. When the tingling is slowed it causes the muscles to rapidly tighten and relax which can help pump blood.

Heat
Heat relaxes muscles, relieves pain, and stimulates blood flow. On the other hand, heat may increase inflammation (swelling) and internal bleeding.

The use of heat can be dangerous. Often a person will put heat on an injury and will feel much better because of the pain relieving and muscle relaxing effect. Underneath, the heat causes the swelling and internal bleeding to increase. After a while the injury is much worse. As a guide, never use heat within three days of doing an injury, or if the injury is still causing sharp or severe pain.

Step two: restoration and rehabilitation

After the swelling has gone down and some of the damage has healed a person will feel much better. Feeling good, patients often think they are fixed. Are they fixed? What do you think?

The answer is no!

The altered balance and movement of the spine will remain. The changes to the muscles, ligaments, discs and so forth that were discussed in chapter nine remain. The abnormal stress on the spine remains.

If left, though the patient may feel good, one or both of the following things are likely.

• The brain will remember which (normal) movement or activity causes the damage, and do its best to avoid that movement or activity. This may be subtle, or something as noticeable as an obvious limp, stoop, or bend.

A patient may remain pain free for a long time doing this, but this limits a person, places abnormal strain on other parts, allows parts to stiffen and deteriorate, and usually eventually causes more serious problems.

• The patient will suffer more pain every time he or she does an activity or movement that aggravates the abnormally stressed areas.

The basic principles of restoration and rehabilitation

To correct the underlying problems in the spine, the changes that are discussed in chapter nine must be reversed. The principles to do this are the same as those for the rehabilitation of an arm that has been broken and wasted away while healing.

First, normal movement must be restored. In the case of the broken arm this is simple - take the cast off. In the case of a spine it is much more complicated, and needs the skillful assistance of a practitioner such as a good chiropractor.

Second, the part must exercise over time to allow the body to restore itself.

The process

Step one: restore movement
In a deteriorated state a spine will not move normally without help. It will much prefer to use parts that are working OK while avoiding using the deteriorated joints.

A skilled practitioner such as a good chiropractor will use specific procedures called adjustments to restore some movement to the abnormal joints.

Because of the deteriorated and changed state of the abnormal joints:
*   normal movement will not be possible at the start, and
*   if left, they will return to their old ways.

After the abnormal joints have had a chance to adapt a bit, but before they fall back into their old ways, the joints are re-adjusted. As this process is repeated full movement is gradually restored.

Step two: strengthening

With full movement restored, the spine can gradually strengthen. During this time the still weakened spine will tend to go back to its old ways, so it will still need regular though less frequent adjusting.

Other forms of care may be needed to support the process. These may include such things as exercises, massage or advice on preventing injury.

The spine originally deteriorated because it was not cared for properly, so once strengthening is finished a sensible maintenance program is recommended to stop similar problems in the future.

Typical spine deterioration

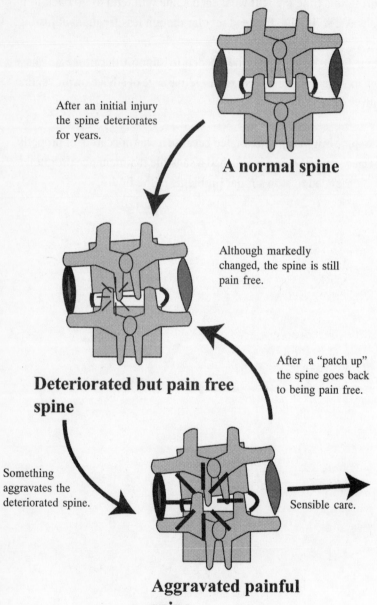

After an initial injury the spine deteriorates for years.

A normal spine

Although markedly changed, the spine is still pain free.

Deteriorated but pain free spine

After a "patch up" the spine goes back to being pain free.

Something aggravates the deteriorated spine.

Sensible care.

Aggravated painful spine

Typical spine restoration

Provided the spine only had moderate muscle and ligamant damage it may restore to near normal.

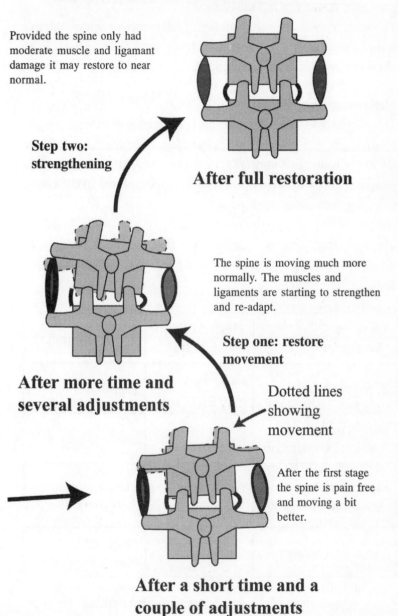

Step two: strengthening

After full restoration

The spine is moving much more normally. The muscles and ligaments are starting to strengthen and re-adapt.

Step one: restore movement

Dotted lines showing movement

After more time and several adjustments

After the first stage the spine is pain free and moving a bit better.

After a short time and a couple of adjustments

How long does the process take?

Step one: Restoring full movement
This varies considerably. Restoration of full movement may be almost instantaneous in a baby or infant, and may not even be possible in an older person with deteriorated joints.

Step two: strengthening
This should be compared to the time taken for a wasted broken leg to return to the same size as the opposite leg. If the leg is in a cast for six weeks restoration may take six months. Most deteriorated spinal joints have been working abnormally for much more than six weeks, so a longer time must be expected.

The following table is a guide. Note that the X-ray changes as discussed in chapter six are used as a guide to the condition of the spine.

Stage of deterioration	Time taken to rehabilitate	What to expect
A normal spine	six to 12 months	full recovery
Mainly muscle and ligament deterioration	one to two years	near normal
Deterioration of the bones and discs also	two to four years	may slow or stop deterioration*
Gross degeneration	Uncertain	keep at it and pray for miracles*

*   Although never as new, they may remain pain free and reasonably servicable. Persons in this condition should learn from the experience and ensure that their children and grandchildren seek appropriate care to prevent the same thing happening to them.

Specific adjustments: the corner stone of the whole process

Adjustments are the corner stone of the whole rehabilitation process. Without them, the spine will never move smoothly and efficiently. Parts of the spine will continue to be overstressed while others waste away. Nerves will continue to be irritated and muscles will continue to tighten.

Why are adjustments so absolutely important?

Lets look at the underlying problem. A spine that has been injured usually has joints that are stiffened or seized, while others are often a little bit sloppy trying to compensate. To make things more complicated, the injured joints may be locked in one direction and sloppy in another.

The practitioner must fully understand spinal movement, and having found the areas of abnormality restore movement using very accurate corrections.

Because they are much easier to learn and to do, many practitioners use gross manipulations instead of adjustments. To a lay person, gross manipulations can be impressive, but they are no where as effective and can be dangerous. See "The difference between a gross manipulation and an adjustment" on pages 122-125.

Treatment of muscles

Often muscles spontaneously recover when adjustments restore normal balance and movement to the spine. Sometimes though they deteriorate enough to become a problem in their own right, and need treatment themselves.

The treatment procedures for muscles are generally straight forward. Some of the basic procedures include the following:

- first aid (rest, ice, compression and elevation),
- massage (or so called 'muscle manipulation'),
- ultrasound and other therapeutic devices,
- stretching, and
- strengthening.

However, for these forms of treatment to be both effective and lasting many things must be ensured.

Muscles must have an un-irritated nerve supply.
If their nerve supply is blocked muscles will not exercise or strengthen properly. If their nerve supply has static they will repeatedly tighten regardless of any stretching or massage.

The joints must be able to move freely.
Unless the joints can move freely the muscles that work them will not be able to exercise (stretch or strengthen) properly.

The spine must be balanced.
If the spine is not balanced muscles will have to work abnormally hard to try and balance it. Despite stretching, massage, and so forth, they will keep tightening.

The tight muscles must not be protecting an injury.
If muscles are tightened to protect an injury loosening them may allow damage, and the muscles will tend to re-tighten.

Muscles must not be compensating for other parts not working.
If they are compensating, the part that is not working needs to be addressed.

The muscles are not restricted by scar tissue or bindings.
If the muscles are restricted by scar tissue or bindings they will not exercise (stretch or strengthen) properly.

The other muscles that work with the muscle must be working normally.
Muscles work together like the instruments in a symphony orchestra. Unless all are working together the finished result is less than optimal.

The body must not have developed subconscious movement patterns that use the muscle abnormally.
If it has, the muscle may not exercise properly, as the body will use the inappropriate movement during exercise.

The muscles must not have any problem that would inhibit it working or be harmed during exercise.
If the muscle has an injury, a very tender tight spot, or some other problem the body may not let it be used. It will instead find some abnormal way to do the movements and activities.

What this all means in practical terms

Most long term problems require some sort of muscle treatment. Unfortunately, many practitioners, such as masseurs, 'muscle manipulators' and other therapists are excellent at what they do, but do not have the educational background to even consider the complex list of questions that must be answered. Therefore, their treatment is often no where near as effective as it could be.

Patients should consult an educated practitioner who specialises in this area, such as a good chiropractor, and follow his or her advice regarding appropriate muscular care.

Prevention

Keep doing the things that injured the spine in the first place and it doesn't matter what the practitioner does, the spine will continue to deteriorate.

Quantum Workhealth, a company that specialises in training workers to prevent injury, showed that it is possible to change unsafe habits provided a person is motivated, given the necessary basic knowledge, and is coached along the way.

Readers will get some idea of what is necessary by reading chapter eight on how a spine is injured. A complete prevention course would take a book on its own. Valuable ideas can often be had from government occupational health and safety material. For example, the Victorian (Australia) government produces an excellent book called the *Manual Handling Code of Practice.*

Exercise

By now the reader will realise that **just** exercising a sore back will not fix the problem. However, exercise as part of a rehabilitation program is an absolute must, just as a previously broken arm must be exercised to regain strength and flexibility.

The choice of exercises is best left to a qualified practitioner who understands the conditions and requirements of a particular spine.

Under general guidelines of the practitioner, qualified gym instructors and other similar professionals are great assets. They are able to advise on exercises and ensure that they are done correctly.

When designing an exercise program the following general guidelines should be used.

1.   Exercise is great for rehabilitation and health maintenance. However, one must be very wary of using exercise as a way of relieving back soreness.

2.   The benefits of exercise are something that cannot be banked. Exercise has to be ongoing. Because of this exercising should be something one enjoys, preferably part of a sport or recreation. If it is not, the exercise will probably only be done until the pain is forgotten.

        However, especially in the early stages of care when the body has gotten used to avoiding using certain parts, very specific exercises may be needed. These should be prescribed by a suitably qualified practitioner who has a specific understanding of the patient's problem.

3.   Someone exercising should be receiving regular checkups from someone qualified in spinal adjusting to ensure that the spine is working normally. If this is not done, the exercises will actually reinforce any problems and cause damage.

4.   When a joint has been stiffened and weakened, no matter how successful an adjustment seems, it will not immediately return to normal. The stiffened, weakened joint can only move so far and do so much.

     If attempting excessive stretching or heavy exercise the body will get the compensating joints to do most of the work.

     On the other hand, exercise that takes the spine through moderate movement with moderate load will likely cause the stiffened, weakened joint to do a reasonable amount of work. Exercises such as swimming and walking for example may cause the stiffened, weakened joint to go through repeated gentle movements, which is ideal.

     As the joint strengthens and frees, the exercise program can gradually get harder.

5.   Given the complex patterns of abnormal balance, movement and compensations that develop in a problem spine, and understanding that the body cannot exercise some deteriorated parts without assistance, one must be extremely wary of any generic exercise program that is claimed to 'fix' back problems.

     Such programs may be found in books or magazines, or even handed out by some practitioners. They often have names such as "spinal mobilisation", "spinal strengthening" or "postural correction".

Step three: maintenance

Why maintenance is needed

After the first two stages of care the patient's muscles, ligaments and spinal movement will be restored as best as possible. In an ideal world the patient would then be able to exercise regularly, avoid bending and twisting, avoid emotional stress, avoid contact sports, plus avoid all the other things that injure a spine, and have no further problems.

This often does not happen. Why?

1. No matter how hard the patient tries there will always be things that injure or upset the balance of a spine. It may be as simple as sleeping with the head on an angle or getting stressed out in a traffic jam, through to a large number of work, sport and leisure related activities.

    Patients don't actually have to "do anything" to upset a the balance and movement of a spine. For example, postural stresses such as poor seating, work postures and standing postures create an abnormal stress. It may be compounded by being overweight or not getting enough exercise.

2. Most patients have some sort of residual damage in their spine. It may be as simple as a bit of scar tissue or fibrosis, through to some roughening of the sliding joints or bony changes. The body will tend to use healthy joints in preference to damaged joints. If the damaged joints are not regularly checked and adjusted they will gradually tighten.

3. As discussed on page 106, it may take years before the spine has fully recovered. Being pain free, it is sometimes assumed that patient's spines are restored and rehabilitated when they are not.

How to maintain your spine

Maintenance is very easy.
* Avoid damaging activities.
* Get regular exercise.
* Have a trusted competent practitioner check and adjust the spine, where necessary, on a regular basis.
* Assess and change any detrimental physical stresses at work, at home, and at recreation or sport.

What will happen at a regular check up?

The patient should feel fine. Often they are surprised when the practitioner finds parts that are still a bit tight or sore, and parts of the spine that do not bend as freely as normal. These are signs that things are not quite right, and there is some underlying stress and damage happening.

The practitioner will help correct the spine.

How regular should check ups be?

A competent practitioner should have a rough idea based on his or her experience with spines in similar conditions.

It is important that the frequency of checkups for a maintenance program be specifically designed for each individual.

Often it may come down to a simple trial and error situation. If maintenance checks are every two months, and the practitioner rarely finds anything to adjust perhaps the interval should be extended. If there are several things that need adjusting maybe the interval needs to be reduced or some different type of care needed.

The false maintenance programs

There are other programs that may be considered to be "maintenance", but are not. It can almost be guaranteed that a patient's spine will continue to deteriorate if adopting these.

Waiting for pain to return
This is also known as "waiting to see how it goes". A patent will stop care until it starts to hurt, then get their spine "fixed" again.

As discussed in chapter five the "fixes" are not real, and as discussed in chapter four the spine can be damaging itself for a long time before it starts to hurt. Underneath the damage will accumulate.

Typically, a person who does this will eventually get to the stage where the problem can't be "fixed", or end up becoming stiff and debilitated.

Waiting till it gets bad enough (or worse, waiting till the pain killers don't work any more)
This is extremely dangerous, but lots of people do it. When they do get bad the problem can be extremely hard to handle, yet the patient will often expect some sort of miracle cure.

Later in life this creates great problems. This is because the accumilated damage is often substantial. It also becomes very difficult to change the old habits that lead to the problem developing.

Chapter Twelve

Extra principles of treatment

Rest and Drugs R.I.P.

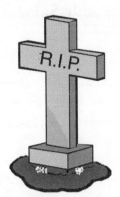

Years ago the mainstay of medical treatment for back pain was simple: rest and take pain killers. In the 1980s some prominent medical specialists started to publish articles with a new message. They realised that prolonged rest and taking pain killers was actually very harmful. While doing very little to help, the prolonged rest would dramatically weaken an already weakened back.

A similar fad existed with the use of neck braces, especially after a motor vehicle accident. While sometimes necessary for a short time when the neck's support structures are badly damaged, prolonged use of a brace quickly causes stiffening and weakening. A patient of this author had actually been placed in a neck brace for eight months. Years later, her head and neck could turn only a little bit each way. Luckily she is still young and with some good care has virtually regained normal movement.

Thank goodness prolonged bed rest and the over use of braces is on the way out.

The latest fad is early exercise and rehabilitation. Though much better than its predecessor, the approach of exercising without adjustments to normalise the spine ignores the fundamental structural, mechanical and neurological changes that have taken place.

What if your Spine is Badly Damaged?

General considerations

Sometimes, the underlying damage is bad enough to create even more serious problems. Examples include a ruptured disc, degeneration, and other substantial damage.

Let's compare these injuries to another well known problem.

A person surviving a heart attack needs to realize two important facts. Firstly, his or her heart is damaged and the arteries are probably clogged with gunk. Secondly, probably years of bad habits such as eating fatty foods and not getting enough exercise caused the problem.

The intensive care department of a hospital may get a heart attack victim past the crisis stage, but the damage and clogging remain. The person will have another heart attack unless he or she realises the limitations imposed by the damages, ceases his or her old unhealthy habits, starts to eat healthily, exercise regularly, and reduce stress levels.

Similar principles apply for a disc injury, degeneration, or other spinal injury with significant damage.

Initial intensive care may get the person out of pain, but the damage and danger remains. Being pain free, patients sometimes believe they are fixed, but relapse is almost certain unless i) the person does things within the limitations imposed by the damage, ii) ceases unsafe practices (see chapter eight), and iii) adopts healthy new habits.

Movement of the damaged joints

Damaged joints will tend to either stiffen or become sloppy.

Stiffening

The body tends to use healthy joints rather than the damaged ones next to them. Used less, the damaged joints will get stiffer and weaker. It's a fact of life. Once damage such as "arthritis" or a disc injury occurs, the joint will need regular adjusting to keep it moving well. Otherwise, it will stiffen, deteriorate and maybe seize.

Sloppiness

A damaged joint may become unstable and slop around with little resistance. When the spine bends most of the movement will be at the unstable joint. This is a nasty situation. The normal joint next to the sloppy one will stiffen and deteriorate. The sloppy joint will try and stabilise itself by growing bone spurs which may grow into a nerve or the spinal cord causing very serious problems.

Managing an unstable joint requires extreme skill and knowledge. For example, it takes great skill to adjust a stiffening normal joint without causing harm by making the unstable joint next to it become sloppier.

Patients whose X-rays show degeneration or bone spurs have a strong possibility of having sloppy spinal joints. They should only have their spines adjusted by a highly qualified practitioner such as a good chiropractor.

The bottom line

Regardless which occurs, a person with a damaged spine needs to be regularly adjusted or the spine will deteriorate much faster than need be.

What a person will feel when the spine is changing back to normal

The most common

Usually after a spine is adjusted a patient will feel a lot better. Feelings of "being freer", "light headedness" and of "being straighter" are very common.

Less common

No matter how gentle and skillful an adjustment is, there is always the possibility of a patient feeling (temporarily) worse afterwards. It is important to know that this is often a sign that good things are happening, and not a reason to worry. This is why.

Minor injury caused by adjustment.
Stuck parts may be held together with scar tissue or adhesions. The scar or adhesions may tear.

The spine doing something new.
Joints or muscles may be doing something they haven't done for years. It's a bit like going for a long run after not exercising for years.

Return of old problems.
There are two main reasons why old problems may return. Firstly, as movement of the spine goes through changes over the years one part may give trouble, then the body learns to compensate and another part starts to give trouble. As the spine is correcting it may go back through the old patterns. This is called "re-tracing".

Secondly, the brain tends to only notice the worst problems. Once these start to go, it focuses on lesser problems (that were there all along). To see how the brain focuses on one problem and forgets others one could find a person with a headache and hit them on the foot with a sledge hammer. It is guaranteed that they would forget all about their headache.

Upsetting the compensations.
When one joint gets out of balance, another will often compensate. When the main problem normalises, the compensation may cause problems until it is corrected.

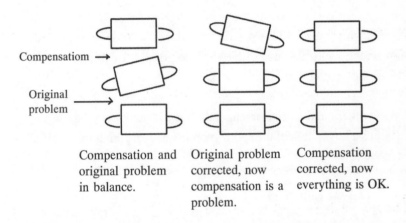

Compensation and original problem in balance.

Original problem corrected, now compensation is a problem.

Compensation corrected, now everything is OK.

Overloading parts that have not healed and strengthened.
With pressure off the nerves, joints moving freely and so forth patients usually feel very good. Sometimes patients feel so good that they forget that their body is still healing and strengthening. Unfortunately when this happens they will sometimes do too much and re-injure themselves.

Sometimes this happens on a sub-conscious level, patients not even realising that they are bending a bit more than they used to, or that a previously stiffened joint is now trying to share some load as more normal movement returns.

The difference between an adjustment and a gross manipulation

As discussed, an injured spine tightens and moves less than it should. Rather than simply the whole spine being stiff, individual joints stiffen while others may move a bit extra to try and compensate. It gets even more complex. Some of the stiffened joints may move freely in some directions while not moving in others.

What they are

An adjustment is a highly specific procedure that restores restricted movement, while placing as little strain as possible on joints that are OK or moving too much.

On the other hand a gross manipulation is a manoeuvre that twists or bends a larger area of the spine, mobilising everything that is able to move.

The skill involved

It takes years of study and practice to give a quality adjustment. To do this the practitioner must thoroughly understand the normal movement of each joint, examine the spine to find abnormalities, and deliver a very accurate correction.

On the other hand, just about any back yard bone cracker or therapist who has done a weekend course can do a gross manipulation. It takes little skill to give someone's spine a good twist until something (or everything) gives.

What they do

An adjustment is a wonderful thing to have done to a spine. The movement of restricted joints is restored gently, without abnormal stress being placed on other parts.

On the other hand a gross manipulation is a horrible thing to have done to a spine. Everything in the area is stretched or traumatised, even the compensating joints that are already sloppy. In the long term, parts may be injured or stretched way beyond their normal limits.

Despite being so bad, a gross manipulation may impress the patient. Some patients feel that the more cracks or the louder they are the better. A manipulation will often make a patient feel better for a short time. In a crude way, it may free up the stiffened joint(s). Any movement where it was previously stiff may relieve pain and muscle spasm.

With the use of gross manipulations, over the years problems usually will keep manifesting. As the years go by the spine deteriorates and may need several gross manipulations to temporarily relieve pain.

Although even a quality adjustment can produce a painful reaction, gross manipulations are much more likely to cause soreness afterwards.

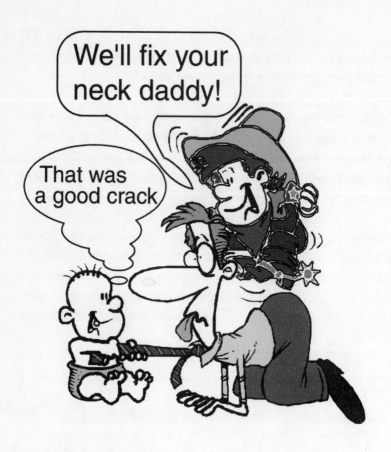

Despite being impressive, loud cracks are not always good for you.

Before   **Adjustment**

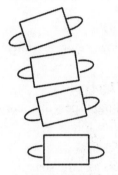 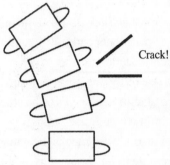

Crack!

One joint stiffened.   Adjustments normalise
the problem.

Before   **Gross manipulation**

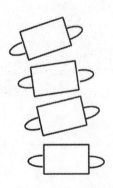 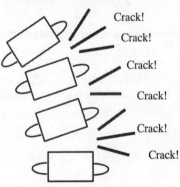

Crack!
Crack!
Crack!
Crack!
Crack!
Crack!

One joint stiffened.   Gross manipulations
crack and traumatise
everything.

How to tell the difference

Unfortunately, it is often hard for a patient to tell the difference between an adjustment and a gross manipulation. Although not absolute, the following list of clues may help.

The manoeuvre is likely to be an adjustment if:
- the practitioner carefully examines the spine before and after each procedure;
- there is only one noise or a small number of noises;
- the practitioner seems to be able to find tight spots that feel painful when pressed upon;
- the practitioner checks the whole spine;
- pressure is felt isolated to only a small area of the spine;
- the practitioner contacts the spine.

The manoeuvre is likely to be a gross manipulation if:
- the practitioner does not seem to thoroughly check the spine before and after each manoeuvre;
- there are a lot of crunches each time it is done, and both sides are 'crunched';
- it feels as though a large area of the spine is being stressed (for example, all of one side of the neck);
- the practitioner only does the painful areas;
- after the first few visits there is still a lot of soreness after each treatment;
- the practitioner does not contact the spine.

Who should you trust to take care of your spine?

The spine is a very complex piece of engineering. To competantly understand how a spine works, how to examine one, and how to treat one, a practitioner really needs a strong background in sciences such as anatomy, physiology, biomechanics and so forth.

Because of this, one should only seek care from a practitioner with a university degree or a similar qualification, and who specialises in this area.

The chiropratic profession has a long and proud background as the leaders in developing the expertise to deal with these problems, and has accumilated a huge body of knowledge. Chiropractors receive a high level of university or college education and many have an approach of treating the cause rather than covering up symptoms.

Though some other practitioners have expertise in caring for spines, the best choice is for patients to seek the care of a chiropractor who uses plans similar to that described within this book, and who has a track record of helping rid patients of pain and helping maintain them in a healthy state.

This book gives the reader a good overview of spinal problems and treatment. It also describes many treatments that are not so good. Patients should ask their chosen practitioner lots of questions and make an informed evaluation.

It gets complicated

Picture this. A joint is injured. A muscle tightens up which pulls another joint out of balance. This causes a nerve to be irritated which effects a muscle a long way away. This throws a further joint out of balance and the chain continues.

It sounds complicated, doesn't it. Consider the following example told by the late master practitioner Dr. A.L. (Roy) Logan, chiropractor from the USA who authored three excellent text books.

Case: Lady with headaches

A lady had headaches. These were relieved for about one hour by adjustments to the neck, for a day by adjustments to the neck and between the shoulder blades, and for a week by adjusting the whole spine and pelvis, but they kept coming back.

In desperation Dr. Logan checked nearly every joint in the body and found a bad problem in a big toe. The patient said "Come to think of it, I stubbed my toe just before the headaches started".

Dr Logan adjusted only the toe. After a short walk the headaches disappeared, never to return.

The more a practitioner looks the more of these patterns are found. Like a chess Grand Master, experienced quality practitioners like Dr. Logan build up a huge database of variations, and can easily solve problems that defy lesser practitioners.

Chapter Thirteen

Special patients and conditions

Children

When do back problems begin? Often it is when someone is being born, falls off the back of the couch, or falls off the swing in the play ground at school. The injured parts lose their normal balance and movement, and the spine deteriorates abnormally.

Those problems are so common that about one in two adolescents have early degeneration visible on a scan of their spine. Many will not get warning signs such as pain for decades. By then the spine may have deteriorated markedly.

If picked up early, these problems can be corrected. Damage and deterioration may be dramatically reduced or stopped altogether.

How can a parent prevent his or her child from developing spinal problems? By far the best way is to have the child regularly checked and examined by a competent professional such as a good chiropractor. This is not unlike having teeth checked regularly for cavities by a dentist.

"Children's adjustments are usually very gentle, and children tend to respond faster to adjustments than adults do."

Infants

The first experience this author had of the awesome effect a spinal complaint can have on an infant was when a worn out mother brought an extremely distressed six month old baby to be checked. For several days the baby had been almost constantly crying, not sleeping for more than one hour at a time. The baby would not even stop crying to feed.

A problem was found in the baby's pelvis. It required only gentle pressure to correct. The baby gave a couple of sighs, then slept for eleven hours. When he woke he was back to normal again.

Scenes like this are repeated in chiropractic clinics every day. In a European trial of over 300 babies with colic over 90% quickly recovered. There were no side effects.

How does a baby's spine get injured?

It's easy. When born, most babies are so weak in the neck that they can't hold their head up. When the mother is pushing to deliver the baby this neck has great pressure on it. As the head comes out it is usually pulled and twisted to get the shoulders through the birth canal.

To see how much a baby's neck can be injured at birth Dr. Towbin of Harvard Medical School examined a lot of still-born babies. In most he found quite a bit of internal bleeding in the neck area, strong evidence of injury.

Another researcher, Dr Frymann, checked 1,250 newborn babies whose births were classified as non traumatic. He found that over three quarters had evidence of neck joint strain.

Checkups

It is sensible for all babies to be checked after birth. As they grow they often do things that potentially injure themselves, so further regular check ups are a must. One only has to understand the slow painless deterioration process that takes place in a spine and that at least 80% of the population end up with bad backs to appreciate the wisdom of regular check ups.

Sick babies

If a baby is sick enough to be of concern he or she should see a suitably qualified practitioner. A sick baby can deteriorate very quickly. If the baby is found to not be in danger there is nothing to stop having the spine checked and adjusted. It is very gentle, very safe, and may be just what is needed.

Colic

Colic literally means that the baby is distressed with apparent stomach pains, but no cause * can be found.

To diagnose colic, a competent practitioner will have checked for the bad things, so this means that the baby is probably in no danger. Standard practices for colic include things such as "doping" the baby with drugs, advising on ways to relieve symptoms, telling the parents that the baby will grow out of it, and even blaming the mother. Because no other cause can be found there is a good chance that the spine may be the problem.

> * As for headaches and other problems caused by interference to the nervous system, medical education and literature tends to either deny or ignore that problems with the spine cause colic. Even if a medical practitioner understood that the spine was a possible cause, baby spines are very small and require genuine skill and expertise to examine, so the examination is best left to someone more appropriately qualified.

Unsettled babies

Often, no cause can be found for babies being unsettled.

What does an adult do when he or she has a problem with the spine and gets headaches, a sore neck or a sore back. They usually feel miserable, whinge and complain. What does a baby do when they get the same problem? Become unsettled??

As with colic, once the baby is cleared of immediate danger get the spine checked out.

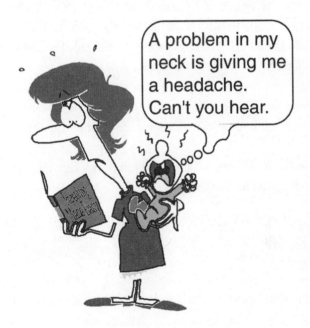

When a baby has a sore neck, sore back
or headache they cannot tell you. They
may just become unsettled and cry.

Older spines

Many older people with deteriorated spines tend to either put up with the pain and stiffness, or take medication such as pain killers or anti-inflammatory drugs. This is often un-necessary and dangerous.

The pain is usually caused by the stiffening and seizing of the joints, and the tightness of the muscles. Stiffened and seized old joints will tend to behave a bit like rusty old hinges. Although it is impossible to restore these joints to like new, often gentle adjusting, muscular work and exercise can restore enough movement to stop pain.

As well, the exercise and increased movement will increase the circulation of blood through the spine and actually improve the muscles and ligaments. The spine will become stronger, and further degeneration will be slowed or stopped altogether.

The combination of removing pain, strengthening, and slowing further degeneration will dramatically improve the person's quality of life.

Because of the deteriorated state of the joints, this care and exercise needs to be regular and ongoing.

Older people should learn from their experiences and encourage their younger friends and relatives to have their spines checked before deteriorating.

Sports

In the sporting area treatment of the spine is often only thought of when an injury occurs. This is the worst way to use quality spinal care.

Optimising performance

Elite level competitions are often won or lost by fractions of a second or very small distances. Even a small problem such as a slightly stiffened joint, a muscle not getting its full nerve supply, or a joint with sensors giving slightly incorrect information can make a huge difference.

Athletes are usually in such good physical condition that their bodies can easily compensate for minor problems. There will be no obvious pain or discomfort. Only a thorough examination (or stop-watch or scoreboard) will pick up the problem.

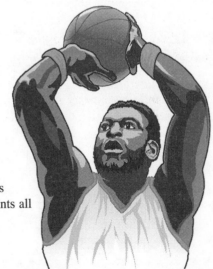

The brain, eyes, nervous system, muscles and joints all working in harmony.

Prevention of injury

Even when an athlete feels all right, there may be some stiffening of joints, tightening of muscles, parts having to do more than their fair share of the work, and so forth. These parts will feel fine normally. When in a competition, straining that last bit or bending that last fraction may cause the overloaded part to give out.

Very simply, if the athlete is kept properly "tuned up" there will be none or very few of those overloaded parts and far fewer injuries.

Treating injuries

When an athlete is injured tuning up the spine can sometimes be like shutting the barn door after the horse has bolted.

Two examples of spinal care being used for sports people and athletes

The injury

Hamstring and groin muscular injuries

How the injury happens

Typically an athlete or player will have abnormal balance or movement of the lower spine. Either through trying to restore balance, trying to protect the spine from damage, or through interference to a nerve, hamstring or groin muscles may become abnormally tight. Often they defy attempts to stretch them.

When competing the abnormally tightened muscles may tear.

Examples of how such injuries can be treated

A poor example
If the lower spine is not recognised as a cause, therapy may be only applied to the damaged muscle. With the cause of tightness remaining the muscle will heal slowly and is likely to tear again when placed under stress.

If the lower spine is recognised as a cause some sort of patch up care is applied. The underlying problem has usually been there for a long time. Given the underlying changes discussed in chapter nine that must be reversed to correct such a problem, and the stress placed on the spine during training and competition, the patch up care will be of little long term benefit.

An excellent example

For athletes to compete at their best they need a medical team including medical doctors, chiropractors, (physical/physio)therapists, trainers, and others all working together for the common good of the patient.

Spinal care, including adjustments where necessary, form part of the pre-season program. Where old injuries are present, a reasonable amount of time will be available before competition for normal balance and movement to be restored, and the muscles and ligaments rehabilitate.

Similar care should be maintained during competition to ensure any injuries and strains retain normal balance and movement as they heal.

By doing this:
- athletes or players will perform better,
- they will be far less likely to be injured, and
- if they do get injured there will be far less underlying structural imbalances, weaknesses and so forth to deal with.
- injury recovery times can be minimised

Training and fitness staff ensure that the players and athletes are fit, and proper warm up and stretching is done before competition.

If an injury does happen treating professionals work as a team. Therapists or other medical personnel may specialise in assisting the muscle to repair, heal and strengthen. During healing, an expert in spinal adjustments can ensure the spine heals with proper balance and free movement.

Similar principles apply to other areas of the body such as the ankles, knees, shoulders and so forth. These joints should be checked and adjusted where necessary to ensure optimum performance and to minimise the chance of injury.

Headaches

One of the most common causes of headache is a problem in the upper part of the spine, usually just below the skull. Either the headache is caused by irritation of the nerves that go up the back of the skull, or the spine refers pain to the head just as a heart attack refers pain to the left shoulder.

When the spine does cause headaches, proper care of the spine usually stops the headaches.

Of course there are many other causes of headaches. Some can be dangerous or life threatening, so it is important to get them checked out by a properly qualified practitioner.

Migraines

Proper migraines are caused by the blood vessels in the head expanding. It is not well known why they enlarge. Stress, light and some foods trigger migraine.

Chiropractors have found that problems with the spine may trigger a migraine to. While a correction of the spine may or may not stop an active migraine, proper spinal care may remove the trigger, and is therefore an excellent preventative measure.

Migraine is often mis-diagnosed, especially by patients. Many "migraines" are nothing more than severe headaches.

Mixed headaches

Most headaches are a bit of a mixture. For example, someone with migraine will tend to become "stressed", and have the neck muscles tighten up. A person with a spinal problem may get "stressed" and end up with a migraine.

The bottom line is that no matter what "label" is put on a headache the spine is often either a cause or becomes involved some way. Therefore, the spine should always be checked by a professional who specialises in this area.

Undiagnosed headaches that are caused by the spine

Despite being arguably the most common cause of headaches, problems with the spine rate scant mention or no mention at all in medical journals or education. Because of this the spine is often not recognised as a cause of many headaches.

What happens when the spine is not recognised as a cause? The following is a composite of many examples seen in clinics around Australia.

Case example: teenager with un-diagnosed headaches

A teenager gets a headache. The medical practitioner examines the patient and finds nothing wrong. Symptom masking drugs are prescribed. The problem persists. More doctors, then eventually specialists are consulted: often neurologists and maybe even a psychiatrist. Expensive tests such as CT scans are done.

By this time the teenager is stressed out and may even be developing psychological problems as well. The parents, having a teenager consulting specialists but still with undiagnosed headaches, will get stressed out. They may even be developing headaches, taking drugs and using medical services as well.

Given the nature of a spinal problem, it will only get worse. In years to come the teenager will be popping arthritis medication as well as pain killers.

The parents may get worried enough to try all sorts of alternative gurus for relief. If lucky, they may stumble across a good chiropractor. Will it then be a happy ending? Maybe, maybe not. Although the problem may have originally been a simple one for the chiropractor, things have changed.

1. The problem in the spine will have worsened considerably.

2. The emotional stress of having a long standing undiagnosed problem will cause a lot of tension and headaches in their own right.

3. Headaches are often a side effect of some headache medications. For example, the sedative/muscle relaxant Diazepam (Valium) has "a hangover like state" listed as a side effect. Headache and dizziness are also listed as side effects for anti-inflammatory drugs including Naproxen (Naprosyn) and Ibuprofen (Brufen).

4. The parents will have become so disillusioned with past failed promises and expectations that they may not persist with the chiropractor long enough for the patient to recover, sometimes even expecting one visit miracles.

Lets be sensible!!

Common sense should be used here. Problems with the spine are a common cause of headaches, while thankfully brain tumours, aneurysms and other dangerous conditions are much rarer.

An excellent person to consult for a headache is a chiropractor. Chiropractors are professionals trained to examine the spine. As well, they are trained to recognise signs of headaches that require other specialised care.

Sciatica

What is sciatica?

Sciatica is pain down the back of the leg, calf and foot*.

What causes sciatica?

The basic principles of spinal injury apply to sciatica. Usually the spine has been working abnormally for years, causing abnormal damage and stress (the condition chiropractors call a subluxation complex). Eventually something gives out causing the pain.

The most commonly understood part to give out is a disc, but there are many other parts that can interfere with a nerve or cause pain down the leg in other ways.

Principles of treatment

As with almost all spinal problems, both the part that gives out and the underlying abnormalities must be taken care of.

Generally, the principles of treatment are exactly the same as those for other spinal problems, as described in chapters eleven and twelve. However, there are two important extra considerations, i) the underlying problem (vertebral subluxation complex) is usually quite substantial, and ii) there may be significant structural damage which the body will be unable to heal itself.

The most significant structural damage is a disc injury.

---

*   Strictly speaking, sciatica is pain caused by irritation to the sciatic nerve which runs down the back of the leg, but sometimes other forms of pain down the leg are labeled 'sciatica' .

Disc injury

A disc injury is a potential disaster!

The outer casing of the disc tears. Like a tyre with a defect in the wall it bulges outward, possibly even rupturing completely.

A word of caution! Even if a bulge is found on a scan, it may not be causing the pain. If 100 "normal" adults were plucked off the street and scanned, about 30 would have disc bulges. Patients with bad sciatica have been treated for a disc bulge, gotten better, yet the bulge was unchanged when re-scanned. Patients who were diagnosed as having a disc injury have had spinal surgery, but the sciatica remains.

The pain down the leg is caused by the disc bulge pressing on a nerve.

Sometimes disc injuries take months and months of frequent expensive treatment to take the pressure off the nerve. Sometimes surgery is necessary.

Even if successful the weakened disc wall means that disc is still only one injury away from disaster. One more injury and the disc may completely rupture or bulge far enough to press permanently on the nerve.

The bottom line for a person with a disc injury is that whatever is necessary must be done to get the pressure off the nerve, then a prolonged process will be needed to correct the underlying problems that cause abnormal stress in the spine. Otherwise, the likelihood of relapse is very high.

Whiplash

What is whiplash?

Whiplash is an injury caused by a severe whipping of the neck, most commonly in a motor vehicle accident.

The often tragic consequence of whiplash

After a whiplash, a patient is usually x/rayed. This is a wise precaution to see if there is severe damage. Usually there is not; often only bruising, swelling, plus some tearing of muscles and ligaments. In this case, the patient is often told that there is nothing seriously wrong, told to rest, given some drugs, a neck brace, and maybe some of the other therapies described in chapter five.

Although bruising and the damage to muscles and ligaments heal in weeks, pain and disability persist. Sometimes years later the patient is re-x/rayed. These x/rays often show a severe deterioration.

To sum up this tragic situation:
- the initial whiplash injury did damage but that damage should heal;
- the injury upset the balance and movement of the spine which causes the spine to rapidly deteriorate for years on.

A sensible approach for whiplash

The patient should be assessed for serious damage, then given a brace and/or any other forms of therapy needed to reduce pain, prevent further damage and assist healing.

In addition, especially once the initial damage has settled a bit, the patient should have his or her spine adjusted regularly to ensure that as it heals it retains normal balance and movement. This dramatically reduces further damage and problems.

Appendix one

Science and back problems

Science is wonderful. It has created many advancements for mankind. The field of spinal care would be very inadequate if not for researchers investigating anatomy, biochemistry, special imaging, pathology, neurology, biomechanics and so forth. Knowledge developed by these people, when combined with intuition and clinical experience, becomes the basis for treatment.

While scientific research and principles are a must, one must be very wary that without a basic understanding and common sense so called science can be used in very misleading ways. How?

It is desirable for treatment to be scientifically tested. In the health care field, the best test is said to be the clinical trial. This is where a group of people receive the test treatment while another group receives a fake or standard treatment. The researchers use some form of measurement to compare the results between groups. The measurement may be as simple as measuring the temperatures or asking whether the person feels better.

This approach is easy when testing say a new drug that lowers temperature. All the researchers have to do is give half the patients the drug and the other half a sugar pill, then measure temperatures.

It is much harder when trying to test treatments for something as complicated as a spinal problem. This is because spinal problems have so many causes and manifestations.

To illustrate how difficult this is, lets examine a well understood problem that also has many causes and manifestations: an overheating car. Causes include a blocked radiator, a burst radiator hose, a broken fan belt, and many more. Manifestations include a glowing temperature light, a loss of power, a cracked cylinder head, steam coming out of the bonnet, and a seized engine.

A competent mechanic would understand how the whole cooling system works, and how to correct the problem. On the other hand, very few spinal care practitioners understand spinal injury and manifestations fully. If car mechanics was structured like the spinal care industry there would be radiator experts, fan belt experts, water pump experts, cracked cylinder head experts, and so forth. To make matters worse, radiator experts would tend to see all overheating problems as being caused by defective radiators. The cracked cylinder head repairers tend to repair cylinder heads not even realising that the fundamental problem may be overheating due to a broken fan belt.

Clinical trials done by spine care people are often very misleading. They can be like getting a large group of overheating cars, replacing the radiators in half, while leaving the other half unchanged, then seeing how many in each group still overheat. Likely, there will only be a few of the overheating cars caused by defective radiators, so only a few will improve. To make matters worse overheating sometimes causes cracks in the cylinder head. Some of the overheating cars caused by defective radiators will have cracked cylinder heads that leak cooling fluid. Fixing the original cause (the radiator) will not stop further overheating.

Clinical trials would show that fixing radiators only worked in a very small number of cars, therefore was not a good way to fix the problem, even though when a radiator is defective it needs replacing.

When vested interests get in the way of common sense, clinical trials can produce some extremely mis-leading results. To illustrate this, lets use a fictitious example to examine the process of a vested interest using clinical trials to market a very ridiculous product.

The company produces a duct that directs cold air from the air conditioner onto the motor, supposedly to reduce overheating. Research facilities such as universities need funds to pay staff, buy equipment, and cover other overheads. A grateful research facility accepts a large dose of cash and agrees to conduct a trial of the ducts.

Half the overheating cars are fitted with the duct, while the other half are not. The cars with the ducts are measured to run on average five degrees cooler. The results are published in the mechanics journal in an article entitled *New Ducting System Causes Overheating Cars To Run Cooler.* The company is able to heavily advertise the ducts as clinically proven products.

Based on this research and publicity mechanics start fitting them!!!

An astute reader may scoff at the preceding example, rightly saying that any intellegent person can see that the ducts from the air conditioner merely cover up the symptom, not fix the cause. They are right, but what do analgesics, anti-inflammatory drugs, and muscle relaxants do???? There have been large numbers of clinical trials on those drugs.

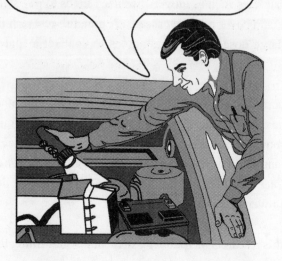

Although obviously ridiculous, a similar thing happens thousands of times each day in "health" clinics.

Science applied to disease caused by the spine

For over 100 years chiropractors have noticed that seemingly un-related problems were cured following adjustments of the spine. These problems include conditions such as indigestion, period pain, asthma, bed wetting, and ear infections.

Armed with the rudimentary science available at the time the chiropractors claimed that bones pressing on nerves caused disease by blocking nerve flow. Removing the pressure from the nerve was said to cure disease. Some chiropractors believed that all disease was caused by misaligned vertebrae in the spine pressing upon nerves.

Since then, science has demonstrated that problems with the spine do irritate nerves, and this can effect the way organs work. Of course, sensible practitioners now realise that there are many different causes of disease.

We now have the situation where on the one hand there are practitioners who see effects of spinal care in practice every day, and on the other hand there are practitioners who will not believe anything until it has been proven in a clinical trial.

The problem is that even if spinal problems caused disease, clinical trials will often not show it. There are two main reasons.

Firstly, like overheating in a car there are often many causes for any condition. For example, indigestion may be caused by a poor diet, emotional problems, diseases of the intestines, and many others.

Lets assume that spinal problems can cause indigestion, and one in ten cases of indigestion are caused by spinal problems. If a trial of 100 people with indigestion was conducted, spinal correction would at best only help about ten people. This would be hard to detect because maybe 10 to 20 people would get better anyway without any treatment.

Secondly, scientific trials like to keep their test treatments simple and standardised, but it has been shown that simple fixes rarely fix anything. In reality, the researchers probably may not even correct the problem in the spine in the first place, so no one will get better from the treatment.

In summary, the basic sciences and clinical experience strongly indicate that spinal problems do cause conditions seemingly unrelated to the spine, and correction of the spinal problem can help. Unfortunately, even if this was quite common, the clinical researchers are unlikely to find it. In the mean time trials continue to supposedly prove the effectiveness of treatments such as analgesics and other drugs, treatments analogous to the previously discussed air conditioning ducts.

A sensible approach seems to be to acknowledge the possibility of a spinal problem as a cause of a disease, and provided there are no serious consequences, have this option investigated by a competent spinal care practitioner.

An even better approach would be to recognise that nerve interference from the spine is detrimental to health, and that the spine should be maintained to enhance health and wellbeing.

Appendix two

How to check if your spine has a problem

The only really effective way to check if your spine has a problem is to have it checked by a professional such as a good chiropractor. Trying to do it any other way is a bit like trying to check one's own teeth for cavities. By the time something shows up there is already a lot of damage.

For those who like to wait until there is a noticeable problem (and a lot of underlying damage), here are some things to look for.

Things one may feel

- Pain in the back or neck
- Pain, numbness or tingling in the arms or legs
- Stiffness
- "Cracks" or grinding" in the spine
- Not able to bend or turn freely
- Headaches
- Dizziness

Things one may notice

- Postural abnormalities (see posture check page 153)
- Obvious stiffness
- Uneven walking
- Weakness in the arms or legs
- Deteriorating athletic performance

Things that may have a spinal cause

- Asthma
- Period pain
- Ear infections
- Bed wetting
- Digestive problems
- Colic or unsettled baby
- Being tired or run down
- Many other seemingly unrelated health problems

Posture check

Probably the best way to check a family member or friend's posture is to look at them from the back. You can pick abnormalities by comparing one side to another.

You can also look from the side. You may look for the head or shoulders being forward, or a "sway back", though it is a bit harder to pick abnomalities because people naturally vary a bit.

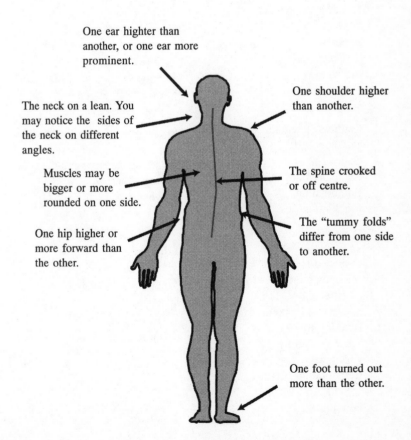

One ear highter than another, or one ear more prominent.

One shoulder higher than another.

The neck on a lean. You may notice the sides of the neck on different angles.

Muscles may be bigger or more rounded on one side.

The spine crooked or off centre.

One hip higher or more forward than the other.

The "tummy folds" differ from one side to another.

One foot turned out more than the other.

Index

www.blcc.com.au

Please check out our web site. You will find a lot more information about different spinal problems and types of treatment.

∨   More information on back care

∨   Answers to common questions.

∨   Send in your own questions to be answered.

∨   Contact the author.

∨   Distributors list

∨   Bulk book orders at very reasonable prices.

∨   Directory of practitioners who provide the type of quality care described in this book.